Infusing
Occupation
Into Practice

Second Edition

Editors

Patricia A. Crist
PhD, OTR/L, FAOTA

Charlotte Brasic Royeen
PhD, OTR, FAOTA

Janette K. Schkade
PhD, OTR, FAOTA

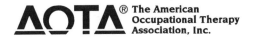
AOTA® The American
Occupational Therapy
Association, Inc.

MT

AOTA Staff

Joseph C. Isaacs, CAE, Executive Director

Chris Bluhm, CPA, CMA, Associate Executive Director, Business Operations Division

Jennifer J. Jones, Director of Publications

Krishni Patrick, MA, Editor, Books

Joyce Raynor, Production Editor

Text design by Robert A. Sacheli, Manager, Creative Services

Cover design by Sarah E. Ely, Book Production Coordinator

The American Occupational Therapy Association, Inc.

4720 Montgomery Lane

PO Box 31220

Bethesda, Maryland 20824-1220

To order call: 1-877-404-AOTA

www.aota.org

Disclaimers

This publication is designed to provide accurate and authoritative information in regard to the subject matter covered. It is sold or distributed with the understanding that the publisher is not engaged in rendering legal, accounting, or other professional service. If legal advice or other expert assistance is required, the services of a competent professional person should be sought.

—*From the Declaration of Principles jointly adopted by the American Bar Association and a Committee of Publishers and Associations*

It is the objective of The American Occupational Therapy Association to be a forum for free expression and interchange of ideas. The opinions expressed by the contributors to this work are their own and not necessarily those of either the editors or The American Occupational Therapy Association.

ISBN 1-56900-107-3

Composition by Circle Graphics, Columbia, Maryland

Printed by Kirby Lithographic Company, Inc., Arlington, Virginia

10/8/03

Table of Contents

Foreword

The Scholarship of Application

The Carnegie Foundation for the Advancement of Teaching identifies four areas of scholarship appropriate for academic institutions: (a) the scholarship of knowledge discovery, (b) the scholarship of teaching, (c) the scholarship of integration, and (d) the scholarship of application (Glassick, Huber, & Maeroff, 1997). The scholarship of application is the use of research and theory in real-life problem setting and problem solving. This current work, the second edition of *Infusing Occupation into Practice*, exemplifies this type of scholarship.

Research and theory have little to offer society unless they are applied and used. Thus, the importance of the scholarship of application is that it applies research and theory in a meaningful way that benefits society. With *Infusing Occupation into Practice, Second Edition,* our goal is to do just that!

For too long, a schism between theory and practice has existed in occupational therapy. Our students are typically well trained in various theories pertaining to occupational therapy. These theories, however, are often relegated to the deep recesses of the therapist's mind when he or she is immersed in the demands of day-to-day practice. The result is a disconnect between theory and practice, a phenomenon common to most practice professions.

To help reduce the disconnection, this edition of *Infusing Occupation into Practice* takes current theories in occupational therapy and applies them to actual cases. This concept, initiated by the Education Special Interest Section under the leadership of Patricia A. Crist, PhD, OTR/L, FAOTA, continues to develop. This edition allows the reader to compare three theoretical views of a given case. It is anticipated that, as with the first edition, this text will be a best-seller and a powerful tool for students, instructors, and clinicians as they link theory to practice.

We give special acknowledgment to Winnie Dunn, Mary Law and David Nelson, the theorists who presented their work at the second Educational Special Interest Section "Infusing" workshop. It is indeed a challenging and daunting process to make theoretical work "real" and "applied" in a way that we can all better access and use. The Education Special Interest Section is an integral part of this ongoing, theory-to-practice process that we hope will continue in future forums. The Education Special Interest Section will host a third workshop at the American Occupational Therapy Association Annual Conference in Philadelphia in 2001.

The mission of the Education Special Interest Section is to foster and strengthen networking among constituents. I truly believe that this book will make a significant contribution consistent with this mission as it provokes spirited and scholarly discussion about theory as operationalized in practice!

Charlotte Brasic Royeen, PhD, OTR, FAOTA

Chairperson, Education Special Interest Section
American Occupational Therapy Association

Reference

Glassick, C.E., Huber, M.T., & Maeroff, G.I. (1997). *Scholarship assessed: Evaluation of the professoriate.* (An Ernest L. Boyer Project of the Carnegie Foundation for the Advancement of Teaching). San Francisco: Jossey-Bass.

Preface

Do not wait for leaders, do it alone, person to person.
Mother Teresa

Every so often, you get the opportunity to observe a transformational moment with far-reaching implications, the collective result of inspirations of a group of colleagues. With the publication of this volume, *Infusing Occupation into Practice, Second Edition,* I feel blessed to have planned and observed the two unfolding Educational Special Interest Section workshops at the Chicago and Indianapolis AOTA National Conferences. The workshops' goal, to provide information and discussion regarding the practical application of various emerging approaches to occupation and the science of occupation, has been expanded with the conversion of these workshops into proceedings that allow wider review and study by practitioners and scholars. As future practitioners, classroom students can also benefit from these proceedings as they see the link between theory and clinical reasoning.

This expanded edition combines the fruits of both workshops. The reader sees the "applied personality" of each approach modeled and analyzed. Through a case study approach, theoretical information about occupation is transformed into practice applications. Presenting two distinct case studies, one from each workshop, allows us to better address the broad spectrum of practice. Dual studies provide an additional resource for students, practitioners, and scholars as they can apply each and work through responses to reinforce their understanding of the application of an approach to practice.

A scholar-to-scholar discussion or debate on approaches to practice is a special event. The true scholar is one who works closely with practitioners to translate their theories and test their work in practice. The greatest gift is when we are encouraged to take the resulting message to fellow professionals and students to enhance the occupational therapy services we deliver. This occurred when a common case study provoked reflection and dialogue that reinforced occupational concepts and illustrated the unique contributions of each approach. This edition includes scholars' comments that give guidance toward the continuing development of their approach through potential clinical and research questions. The interaction between practice and research breathes "life into theory." The result is that information regarding "best practices" emerges to be shared.

To prepare these extended proceedings for publication, each presenter was asked to retain the natural discourse context within his or her workshop sections as much as possible. Each presenter lightly edited his or her taped and transcribed presentation. This monograph includes the visual materials used during the workshops. In this expanded edition, three new approaches were added to the original three, and the authors of the first edition were invited to write a brief piece reflecting on the development of their approach over the past four years. We believe that these proceedings capture the essence of six scientists' work from a pragmatic perspective.

The seamless integration of occupation into our professional core for occupational therapy is essential. The scientific study and application of occupation are tantamount to occupational therapy being fully recognized as a profession. This monograph captures a historical moment and brings science to our practice. Fretting over health care changes does not alter the conditions for practice—we can only do so through the choices we make in our practice. In closing, I am reminded of Helen Keller's words: "When one door of happiness closes, another opens; we often look so long at the closed door that we do not see the one which has opened for us."

Here is your open door. No need to knock! Come on in and reflect awhile on the contents of *Infusing Occupation into Practice, Second Edition.*

Patricia A. Crist, PhD, OTR/L, FAOTA
Senior Editor

Acknowledgments

The editors would like to thank Mary Jane Snyder for her excellent transcription, communication with authors, and preparation of the final draft of this manuscript. Not vacations, computer viruses, or our last-minute request thwarted her from this task. Her insight was exemplary as she translated spoken words and imagined personalities into a written format that captures the character of an important historical moment in our profession. By using a technology system she established, we were able to quickly bring this publication to fruition. Ms. Snyder has been instrumental in the creation of both the first and second editions of *Infusing Occupation into Practice*.

The EDSIS Standing Committee gratefully thanks Drs. Sally Schultz, Gary Kielhofner, and Florence Clark for participating in the first workshop in Chicago, and David Nelson, Winnie Dunn, and Mary Law for participating in the second workshop in Indianapolis. Through this work, they have demonstrated unselfish servant leadership in making the initial, invited presentation at the AOTA Annual Conference and Expositions and in helping review the transcribed proceedings to create this monograph.

Infusing Occupation Into Practice

Workshop sponsored by the Education Special Interest Section of the American Occupational Therapy Association at the 1996 Annual Conference and Exposition, April 19–23, 1996 in Chicago, Illinois.

Presenters

Occupational Science

Florence Clark, PhD, OTR, FAOTA
Professor and Chair, Department of Occupational Therapy
University of Southern California

Model of Human Occupation

Gary Kielhofner, DrPH, OTR/L, FAOTA
Professor and Head, Department of Occupational Therapy
University of Illinois at Chicago

Occupational Adaptation

Sally Schultz, PhD, OTR
Associate Professor, School of Occupational Therapy
Texas Woman's University

Editors

Patricia A. Crist, PhD, OTR/L, FAOTA
Chair and Professor, Department of Occupational Therapy
John G. Rangos, Sr. School of Health Sciences,
Duquesne University

Charlotte Brasic Royeen, PhD, OTR, FAOTA
Assistant Dean of Research, Professor of Occupational Therapy,
School of Pharmacy and Allied Health Professions, Creighton University

Theoretical References

Occupational Adaptation

Garrett, S., & Schkade, J. K. (1995). Occupational adaptation model of professional development as applied to level II fieldwork, *American Journal of Occupational Therapy, 49,* 119–126.

Schkade, J. K., & Schultz, S. (1992). Occupational adaptation: Toward a holistic approach for contemporary practice, part I. *American Journal of Occupational Therapy, 46,* 829–837.

Schultz, S., & Schkade, J. K. (1992). Occupational adaptation: Toward a holistic approach for contemporary practice, part II. *American Journal of Occupational Therapy, 46,* 917–925.

Model of Human Occupation

Helfrich, C., & Kielhofner, G. (1994). Volitional narratives and the meaning of therapy. *American Journal of Occupational Therapy, 48,* 319–326.

Munoz, J., Lawlor, M., & Kielhofner, G. (1993). Use of the model of human occupation in psychiatric practice. A survey of skilled therapists. *Occupational Therapy Journal of Research, 13,* 117–139.

Occupational Science

Yerza, E. J., Clark F., Frank, G., Jackson, J., Parham, D., Pierce, D., Stein, C., & Zemke, B. (1989). An introduction to occupational science, a foundation for occupational therapy in the 21st century. *Occupational Therapy in Health Care, 6*(4), 1–17.

Clark F. A., Parham, D., Carlson, M. E., Frank, G., Jackson, J., Pierce, D., Wolf, R. J., & Zemke, R. (1991). Occupational science: Academic innovation in the service of occupational therapy's future. *American Journal of Occupational Therapy, 45,* 300–310.

Clark F., Carlson, M., Zemke, R., Frank, G., Patterson, K., Larson, B., Rankin-Martinez, A., Hobson, L., Crandall, J., Mandel, D., & Lipson, L. (1996). A qualitative study of the life domains and adaptive strategies of low-income well elderly. *American Journal of Occupational Therapy, 50,* 99–108.

Clark, F. (1993). The 1993 Eleanor Clarke Slagle Lecture: Occupation embedded in a real life: Interweaving occupational science and occupational therapy. *American Journal of Occupational Therapy, 47,* 1067–1078.

Note from the Editors

While planning this workshop, the three presenters worked from two different versions of the case study. In one, the individual was described as having a significant problem with alcohol. In the later version of the case study, this problem was not emphasized. Accordingly, the comments may vary.

In preparing the proceedings, each presenter was asked to retain the natural discourse context from the original proceedings as much as possible. The contributors were permitted to edit their own sections before publication, thus accounting for some variance in the discourse presented here.

The appendices were created to permit each presenter to publish visual material used during that person's presentation or to add information when preparing this monograph. As a result, these proceedings "capture the moment."

In the theoretical references, each author cites the two to four works that provide the reader with an introduction to the approach discussed.

Introduction

Patricia Crist

Welcome to Workshop B-1 of the Education Special Interest Section. We will be discussing "putting occupation back into education and practice." I am very pleased to have this illustrious panel gathered here at one time and place to discuss a common case study. I would like to share with you that Charlotte and I dreamed about the need to clarify the framework for occupation about 3 years ago. One of the things we realized is that practitioners, both in education and in the clinical areas, were seeing the work of occupational adaptation, occupational science, and model of human occupation emerge in many different but separate ways through professional writings, in meetings, and in various other discussions. What was missing was a comparison of the three approaches from a common clinical perspective. We have invited three individuals who are the leaders in developing each of these approaches to present to you, and give us an opportunity to talk about, the similarities and differences when discussing and focusing on one common clinical case. I am very excited that we're experiencing this event together, and I look forward to hearing the information they are going to impart to us.

I would now like to take the opportunity to introduce to you Dr. Charlotte Royeen, who will be the moderator for the panel today and who was my codreamer about 3 years ago, when we first thought of bringing these folks together. Dr. Royeen is at Shenandoah University,[1] where she has implemented a new educational program.

I do not want to take any more time, as I know you would rather hear the speakers. So let us begin!

Charlotte Royeen
Moderator

My charge today is to keep temporal order on three of the best brains in the world. I will be the "temporal order-keeper." I am setting the ground rules now, and after the ground rules, we will have warmups for each speaker, allowing each of them 10 minutes to present the key concepts underpinning their theories. After the key concepts are presented, we'll take a moment and you can read through the case. Following your reading of the case, each of the panel members will take the first question on the case and have a 5-minute discussion of it. Then we will go to the second question,

---

[1] At the time of the workshop, Dr. Royeen was working as a program director at Shenandoah University in Winchester, VA.

and each panel member will present a 5-minute discussion. Then we will do the third question, and so on.

Finally, each panel member will have an opportunity to link his or her theory to education and practice, which is our primary goal for this EDSIS workshop. At the end, we will entertain general questions. I suggest that while the presentation is going on, if burning questions occur to you, please jot them down so that when we come to the question-and-answer period, you will be ready.

I think these speakers need no introduction. If you look at the brochure for "Back to the Future in Occupation," you will see the pedigrees presented for Dr. Sally Schultz, Dr. Gary Kielhofner, and Dr. Florence Clark. Again, I want to extend a personal thanks to all of them for sharing their expertise in this format. The current workshop format is something that is new to us, and it is quite extraordinary that Drs. Schultz, Kielhofner, and Clark were willing to spend the time and the energy preparing for the workshop on such short notice. This format is very challenging for speakers and we thank these three for their commitment to education.

Overview of Theoretical Models

Occupational Adaptation

Sally Schultz

I would like to preface my remarks with this statement: "The artist who really creates something, creates it forever, but the scholar is at the mercy of expanding knowledge and changing habits of thought" (quote is credited to C. M. Bowra, born 1898—location of citation unknown). It is in this spirit that I invite your scrutiny of what I present to you today. I will present the key concepts and the assumptions that I believe define the boundaries for occupational adaptation.

First of all, occupational adaptation is a frame of reference that has been developed for use in practice. Its function is to guide the practitioner's thinking and decision making and to generate the critical questions the practitioner must ask. The answers will always be unique to the individual being treated. When Janette Schkade and I began to formulate these ideas on occupational adaptation, our discussions were based more on our understanding of practice than on any particular theoretical perspective. The foundation for this frame of reference represents an integration of two of the professions' most enduring concepts—*occupation* and *adaptation*. Our understanding of occupational adaptation provides the boundaries that delineate this frame of reference. In the remainder of my remarks, I will present the essence of those boundaries.

To begin, my frame of reference is the normative process that underlies the phenomenon of human adaptation and how that adaptation is affected by occupations. Five key concepts are identified in today's presentation (See Appendix A: Occupational Adaptation). The term *occupation* must be specifically defined within this frame of reference. We define occupation as "those activities in which the individual has active involvement; experiences personal meaning; and engages in a process that yields a product, either tangible or intangible."

We also need to define *adaptive response*. The adaptive response is the internal mechanism that the individual activates to create a plan of action that responds to an occupational challenge. The occupational challenge is a difficulty or dilemma that the individual experiences in response to demands for occupational performance. The term *occupational environment*, as specifically defined in this frame of reference, describes the physical, social, and cultural context in which work, play, and self-maintenance performance occur. Thus, occupational challenges are embedded in the individual's interpretation of the occupational environment and his or her respective role.

Three constants form the occupational adaptation process. They are (a) the person's desire for mastery, (b) the environment's demand for mastery, and (c) the resulting press for mastery. These constants are the source of the occupational performance demands and the resulting challenges. Their interplay calls forth an internal adaptive response, which sets the stage for the resulting occupational response. The *occupational response*, then, comprises the observable behaviors or actions that occur as a result of the occupational challenge.

The final concept I will introduce is called *relative mastery*, which also is specific to the occupational adaptation frame of reference. Relative mastery is defined as "an evaluation of the occupational response that is made by the individual and based on personal standards." Thus, mastery in occupational adaptation is always perceived as relative.

The individual uses three conditions to evaluate relative mastery. They are (a) the degree of efficiency experienced, (b) the degree of effectiveness, and (c) the satisfaction to self and society.

We believe that these normative concepts articulate a rationale for occupational therapy intervention that is specifically directed at the individual's internal process of adaptation. That process is the target of therapy within this frame of reference.

What modality is used? Clearly, occupation is the most powerful tool the therapist has. First, occupation will readily tap into the client's personal mechanism of adaptation. Second, occupation is the most effective way to promote improvement in the client's ability to adapt in ways that will maximize the experience of relative mastery. The interventions used in occupational adaptation are basically one of two forms of occupation. Each will be briefly discussed as follows:

1. *Occupational readiness*—techniques used to treat sensorimotor, cognitive, and psychosocial impairments. The form that readiness takes must be directly linked to the occupational environment and the respective role that the client has selected as most significant.

2. *Occupational activity*—tasks that meet occupational adaptation's definition of occupation, mentioned earlier, and that are part of the occupational environment, plus the respective role the client has selected for focus in therapy.

Sally Schultz

An occupational adaptation approach demands a therapeutic relationship that is process oriented, wherein the client is acknowledged as the agent of change. The therapist is recognized as the client's facilitator. This recognition is accomplished by engaging the client in occupation-based experiences that call for an adaptive response. The therapeutic process becomes one in which the therapist is developing the client's adaptiveness rather than helping the client adapt.

Model of Human Occupation

Gary Kielhofner

The model of human occupation grew out of Mary Reilly's occupational behavior tradition at the University of Southern California. I remain indebted to her thinking and mentoring. Over the past 21 years, this model has been expanded, researched, revised and applied by many people. It has been my privilege to work with such sound thinkers and researchers as Janice Burke, Roanne Barris, Ann Fisher, and Alexis Henry, who have made important contributions to this model. I am indebted to an international group of persons who contributed significantly to the model's development, in particular, Hans Jonsson and Lena Borell, along with other Swedish colleagues at Stockholm University and the Karolinska Institute. Finally, over the past decade my colleagues at the University of Illinois at Chicago have also greatly influenced the development of this model. Chris Helfrich, Jaime Muñoz, Trudy Mallinson, Craig Velozo, and too many others to mention have been very important collaborators.

To be asked to summarize more than 2 decades of work in 10 minutes is not unlike torture. However, I will do my best to briefly characterize the model's arguments and concepts, referring mainly to what is published in the second edition of *A Model of Human Occupation: Theory and Application* (Kielhofner, 1995). I will summarize the model in six theoretical arguments presented in Table 1.

Three Subsystems

The first argument is that the human being is a complex organization of three subsystems: volition, habituation, and mind-brain-body performance. These subsystems respectively motivate, organize, and make possible the performance of occupation. We propose that it is the role of volition to choose occupational behavior, the role of habituation to organize occupational behavior into the patterns necessary for one's lifestyle, and the role of the mind-brain-body performance subsystem to support skilled performance.

Interaction of Human and Environment

The second argument is that occupational behavior emerges from the interaction of the human system with the environment. We further assert that occupational behavior shapes the subsequent

Table 1. Theoretical Arguments of the Model of Human Occupation.

---

1. The human being is a complex organization of three subsystems (volition, habituation, and mind-brain-body performance) that motivate, organize, and make possible the performance of occupation.

2. Occupational behavior emerges from interaction of the human system with the environment. Further, occupational behavior shapes the subsequent organization of the human system.

3. The volition subsystem arises from a need for action and is composed of personal causation (beliefs and feelings about one's capacity and control), values, and interests. This subsystem anticipates, chooses, experiences, and interprets occupational behavior.

4. Occupational behavior demonstrates a pattern that is influenced by one's habituation subsystem; this subsystem is composed of habits and internalized roles.

5. Occupational performance is composed of motor, process, and communication/interaction skills, which emerge from the interaction of one's mind-brain-body performance subsystem with the environment.

6. The social environment (including occupational forms and social groups) and the physical environment (including objects and spaces) provide both opportunities and constraints, which shape occupational behavior.

---

organization of the human system. Consequently, we view human beings as dynamic, self-organizing systems that spontaneously assemble their behavior in real time within an environmental context. As human beings engage in work, play, and daily living tasks, they also shape and change their own organization by reinforcing, elaborating, and altering dimensions of the self, such as capacities, beliefs, and dispositions.

Volition System

The third argument states that *volition* arises from a need for action and is composed of personal causation, values, and interests. This subsystem anticipates, chooses, experiences, and interprets occupational behavior. The human need for action is uniquely expressed in each person's *activity choices,* which are decisions about the use of discretionary time in everyday life, and in *occupational choices,*

Gary Kielhofner

through which persons select the roles and habits that constitute their lifestyles.

Volition emerges and changes through occupational behavior. As people act in the world, they accumulate a sense of (a) their own effectiveness and awareness of potentials for enjoyment, (b) potentials for satisfaction, and (c) a view of life that commits them to behave in certain ways. These areas of self-awareness are referred to, respectively, as personal causation, values, and interests.

Personal causation includes one's knowledge of capacity (i.e., an awareness and an attitude toward one's present and potential abilities) and one's sense of efficacy (i.e., the perceptions of one's command of personal behavior and of one's effectiveness in achieving desired outcomes).

Values are a coherent set of convictions that assign significance or standards to occupations, creating in each person a strong disposition to perform accordingly. *Personal convictions* refer to one's way of viewing life and the goals to be pursued in life. These convictions are, simply, commonsense beliefs about what matters in life. These views generate commitments or strong emotional dispositions to follow what are perceived as the right way to behave.

Interests are dispositions to find pleasure and satisfaction in occupations, coupled with the self-knowledge of this enjoyment of occupations. The disposition to enjoy certain occupations and certain aspects of performance is referred to as *attraction*. Attraction to any particular occupation ordinarily represents a confluence of several factors, such as enjoying the challenge, aesthetics, products, or human interaction provided by that occupation. *Preference* refers to the configuration of one's favored occupations and way of acting.

Volition is, above all, an active process of participating, choosing, experiencing, and interpreting one's occupational behavior. Volitional thoughts, feelings, and choices reverberate with present circumstances, past memories, and images of a possible future. People integrate their past, present, and future into a coherent whole that we call *volitional narratives*. These are very highly personal life stories: Within the volitional narrative, an individual makes sense of his or her own competence and considers how to find satisfaction and value in life. Through their occupational behavior, people strive to continue the volitional narrative in ways that they believe are important, that bring satisfaction, and that are seen as achievable.

More importantly, not only do narratives influence how we actively experience and interpret our occupations, but also they influence how we select and organize our behavior. We choose and engage in occupations as an act of living our narratives. Hence, the motivation for occupation involves both an active telling and an active behaving of our volitional narratives.

Habituation Subsystem

The fourth argument is that occupational behavior demonstrates a pattern influenced by the habituation subsystem. This subsystem is composed of habits and internalized roles. To be competent, people must be integrated into the rhythm and customs that make up their physical, social, and temporal worlds. Moreover, people move through life occupying a sequence of social positions. The process of acquiring and repeating these patterns of occupational behavior is referred to as *habituation*.

Habituation is a dynamic process in which internalized roles and habits allow us to appreciate and cooperate with our familiar and recurrent temporal, physical, and social environments. Habits and roles are not instructions for behavior. Rather, they are tacit frameworks from which we encounter and traverse our world. Finally, habituation is a self-organizing process by which the very behaviors that habituation evokes will serve to sustain habituation.

Habits preserve our ways of doing things that we've learned from earlier performance. Once in place, habits allow behavior to unfold almost automatically. Habits organize occupational behavior by (a) influencing how one performs routine activities, (b) regulating how time is typically used, and (c) generating styles of behavior. The *internalized role* is a broad awareness of a particular social identity and related obligations, which together provide a framework for appreciating situations and constructing behavior. Roles influence (a) our interactions with others, (b) the kinds of tasks we perform, and (c) the way we partition time.

Mind-Brain-Body Subsystem

The fifth argument is that occupational performance is composed of motor, process, and communication and interaction skills. These skills emerge from the interaction of one's mind-brain-body performance subsystem with the environment. We conceptualize skill as distinct from capacity. *Capacity* refers to the underlying potential for behavior, but *skill* refers to the characteristics of actual performance.

Social and Physical Environment

The sixth assertion is that the environment, including occupational forms, social groups, physical spaces, and objects, provides both opportunities and constraints that shape occupational behavior. The environment does this in two ways, by *affording* or giving opportunities for performance, and by *pressing*, which means to recruit or demand particular behavior.

Gary Kielhofner   Social groups include enduring collections of people, such as a family or work colleagues, and temporary gatherings, such as this morning's workshop. Every group has its own dynamic conditions that influence behavior. *Occupational forms* (a concept based on Nelson's [1988] work) refers to coherent sets of actions that are oriented to a purpose or goal and that are generated and sustained in the social collective. The physical environment includes natural and fabricated spaces (e.g., parks, rooms, fields, paths, hallways, ponds, closets) and objects (e.g., eggs, apples, nuts, knives, forks, plates).

Groups, occupational forms, spaces, and objects coalesce into coherent environments that we refer to as *occupational behavior settings*. Occupational life involves passage through and interaction with a series of occupational behavior settings that include home, school or workplace, neighborhood, and recreation and resource sites, such as stores and theaters.

In summary, the model of human occupation views the human being as a dynamic self-organizing system that exists and acts in relationship to a physical, temporal, and social environment. The model attempts to address (a) how people are motivated to choose, experience, and interpret their occupations; (b) how occupational behavior is organized into the patterns that make up everyday life; and (c) how performance is constructed. The model emphasizes the centrality of occupational behavior in shaping the organization of the human being. It emphasizes process over structure, calling attention to occupation as the process (a) by which we take hold of, and are influenced by, the world around us; (b) by which we fill our days with action; and (c) by which we fashion ourselves into the beings we are becoming.

Occupational Science

Florence Clark   Before I discuss the key components of the occupational science perspective, I will address what occupational science is and how it can relate to practice. To begin with, occupational science is an academic discipline, as is sociology or psychology (Appendix C: Occupational Science, Table 1). Occupational science is concerned with the study of the human as an occupational being. It is not conceived of as a frame of reference for treatment. It is not a frame of reference! It does not contain established guidelines for treatment or a prepackaged format for treating patients. However, individual practitioners may draw from knowledge generated in occupational science to inform their clinical reasoning about specific cases. At the University of Southern California (USC), oftentimes, what we do as we delve into the knowledge base of occupational science is to conjecture on how what we are reading relates to practice. We often try to think about what treatment would look like if it were derived or guided by some of the ideas contained in whatever we are reading. Thus, what I am going to present today are my thoughts on this case, which are combined with the opinions of eight USC occupational science doctoral students and which are based on a circumscribed set of readings we were studying in a seminar. The PhD students are Don Gordon, Deborah Mandel, Renee McDannel, Ann McDonald, Phyllis Meltzer, Brenda Scroggins, Susan Spitzer, and Brian Young, all of whom were in a course that I taught this semester and in which we worked on the case presented here today. Appendix C: Occupational Science, Table 2 lists the books that guided our thoughts on the case. It is crucial that you realize that if we had been reading other books, we might have come up with a completely different conceptualization of how we would treat the case. The perspective I am presenting is one that emerged from our synthesis of the specific ideas that were relevant to occupational science and that were contained in this set of books.

However, our analysis was also influenced by certain broad assumptions of occupational science that are listed in Appendix C: Occupational Science, Table 3. The first fundamental assumption is that engagement in meaningful occupation is essential to health; the second is that there is a recursive relationship between occupation and narrative that shapes personal identity. Perhaps some of you saw Pollie Price-Lackey's article (Price-Lackey & Cashman, 1996) in the most recent issue of the *American Journal of Occupational Therapy*. The article described the recovery of Jenny Cashman and discussed the recursive relationship between narrative and occupation. This relationship means that narrative imbues occupation with meaning, but as we engage in occupation, we are revising our narratives or our understanding of the world and of ourselves. Humans construct their identities; they create their sense of self as they engage in meaningful and satisfying occupations. The third assumption is that humans are most true to themselves when they are engaged in meaningful and satisfying occupations.

In Appendix C: Occupational Science, Table 4, I have listed the key concepts that were derived from the readings (Appendix C: Occupational Science, Table 2) and that formed the basis of our thinking about this case. First, by examining Foucault (see Rabinow, 1984), we extracted the idea of resistance to disciplinary practices and the need to counteract the medical model. Foucault is a postmodern philosopher who has written about how particular disciplinary practices in our culture serve the interests of power structures.

Florence Clark

For example, he suggests schools may be part of a disciplinary structure that creates docile bodies. One way in which schools accomplish the molding of children into docile bodies is by enforcing a particular time schedule. You may remember that in your own school experience the bells would ring at 8:05, and at that time you would have to go to your first class. Another bell would ring 45 minutes later and you were trained to go to recess. Schedules create docile beings who respond to bells and schedules, the kind of people who would be good factory workers. So Foucault sees normal schools as serving the interests of industrialized societies that need to train people to work as laborers in factories. I cannot, of course, cover Foucault's ideas in any depth in this brief presentation, but our group felt that we needed to look at disciplinary practices. Foucault describes classification, categorization, and punishment as the methods that power structures use to enforce conformity. Our group was inspired to think about this case in terms of Foucault's idea of resistance to disciplinary practices.

Second, drawing on Kondo (1990), we believed it was important to think about how different selves are constructed through occupation in the context of one's life, and to think in terms of selves instead of roles. We rejected the notion of thinking in terms of role dysfunction, because on the basis of Jackson (unpublished manuscript, 1993), we adopted the view that role emphasizes conformity, consensus, and compliance with social norms. Role does not tend to sanction nonconventional, individualistic solutions to problems in life. We played with the idea that the concept of *match* might be more useful than the concept of *role* in thinking about this case. We examined the case of a teenage girl who allegedly had an occupational role dysfunction while attending a school for girls, but who, once she transferred to another school, began to flourish because of the match between the structure of the new school and her needs. The expectations of the first school's culture did not fit the particular attributes that this individual had at the time. By her simply switching environments, what one might conclude to be an occupational role dysfunction was eliminated. Our group, therefore, chose to address in Dee's case the concept of different selves as crafted in different situations and settings.

Third, we believed we needed to consider the patient's system of meaning: one's narrative interpretation of one's self as an occupational being must be the centerpiece of treatment. In the interest of time, I will not say much about this concept, but for those who are not familiar with it, I have covered it extensively in my Slagle lecture (Clark, 1993), and I believe many of you are quite familiar with my thoughts on this concept.

Fourth, we decided to work with the notion that meaningful occupation possesses powerful transformative potential. This idea comes from the anthropological studies of Turner (1987), as does the fifth concept we chose to think about in addressing this case, that patients may be viewed as protagonists in a social drama. *Social drama* is defined by Turner as a crisis in which some breach has occurred and in which there is a need to redress the situation. As therapists, we can think about case studies in terms of what type of interruption or breach has occurred in a person's life. We can ask what can be done to redress the situation. Our group used this idea of social crisis and breach as a way of thinking about this case.

You must remember that this orientation and the theoretical concepts I have just listed are unique to the particular body of literature (see Appendix C: Occupational Science, Table 2) that we were reading in a particular class—a class that I was teaching at the time I was invited to think about this case study. Had our group been reading other books, I believe our approach, while sharing some commonalities with what I am presenting today (for example, a focus on the human as an occupational being), might have been quite different in other ways.

Case Study: Dee Jackson*

Dee Jackson is a 33-year-old, separated, female who has served in the U.S. Army (E–5) with 11 years of continuous active duty. In July 1991, she was diagnosed with a major depression, placed on antidepressant medication, and initially admitted to the acute psychiatric ward at an Army medical center. The course of events preceding her admission were vague and unusual. While Sergeant Jackson was completing a tour of duty in Saudi Arabia, her husband spent their life savings and turned their children over to her mother for care. When she returned to the United States, Sergeant Jackson had difficulty coping and was admitted to a civilian hospital for 2 months. After hospital administrators realized Sergeant Jackson was on active duty, they sought transfer to a military hospital.

In August 1991, Debbie Sanders, OTR, interviewed Sergeant Jackson. At that time, Ms. Sanders' impression was that Sergeant

---

*Dee Jackson is a case study that has been adapted from a narrative prepared by Nedra Gillette during the clinical reasoning studies sponsored by the American Occupational Therapy Foundation (AOTF).

Jackson was experiencing an occupational role disruption that was secondary to several lifestyle stressors. Sergeant Jackson reported she had entered the military directly from high school as an administrative clerk, her military occupational specialty. At one point, however, Sergeant Jackson stated she had worked for a limited time with the U.S. Postal Service. While she identified that she valued her role as a mother, Sergeant Jackson remained unable to sort out the frustration and confusion she had experienced since her return from Saudi Arabia. In addition, she identified a pattern of maladaptive behavior that had started before her marriage. Throughout the interview Sergeant Jackson focused on her experience in Saudi Arabia, and was unable to address any future issues or concerns.

During her initial stay, Sergeant Jackson progressed in the ward status system, but conflicting medical appointments often caused sporadic attendance in occupational therapy groups. The initial conference for planning a multidisciplinary treatment determined that Sergeant Jackson's condition did not warrant a medical discharge from the military. She was expected to remain on the ward for a short stay and to return to her unit for administrative action once the psychotic features were no longer an issue. Approximately 10 days following the initial treatment planning conference, her team met a second time because Sergeant Jackson seemed to regress every time she was faced with returning to her unit. Knowing that Sergeant Jackson would receive limited compensation, the physician decided to proceed with a medical evaluation board. The team decided to focus on her lack of insight, poor work performance, and sporadic attendance at treatment groups.

During occupational therapy treatment groups, Sergeant Jackson was manipulative, attempting to be removed from groups. At the objection of the occupational therapy department, Sergeant Jackson was placed on 2 weeks' leave for the purpose of returning to her family to attend to business. On her return, Sergeant Jackson was transferred to a limited-care ward that focused on transition into civilian life. She managed to assimilate the demands of the limited-care ward for approximately 2 weeks before she was transferred back to the acute-care ward with a DSM III-R diagnosis of post-traumatic stress disorder and alcohol abuse with depression.

When she returned to the acute-care ward, Sergeant Jackson was placed on restricted status that did not permit her to attend off-ward activities, so she received occupational therapy services on the ward. She reported hearing voices and experiencing an increase in nightmares that told her to harm herself. At that time, she was focusing on her failure and her desire to "kill herself" as the answer to her problem. During the course of her hospitalization on the acute psychiatry ward, Sergeant Jackson was followed by occupational therapy practitioners, who found her a difficult patient: she was unable to concentrate on tasks for any length of time and she remained focused on suicide as her only answer. Additionally, Sergeant Jackson did not appear to invest in activities for her children or for others. Occupational therapy practitioners continued to include Sergeant Jackson in groups that would assist her in the future; however, she provided only minimal input into this process. On her discharge Sergeant Jackson was transferred to a Veterans' Administration hospital, near her mother and children, for additional treatment.

Case Study Questions

1. Based upon your theoretical reference, how do you begin to understand this person? How do you assess and evaluate or understand function/dysfunction?

2. Based upon your theoretical reference, how would you begin the intervention process? Or, how would factors influencing the unfolding of the person's story be considered?

3. Based upon your theoretical reference, what are projected outcomes for this person?

4. What research questions are viable or needed to study clinical application of your work?

Case Study Discussion

Charlotte Royeen

This interactive case has had various forms in life. The case study of Dee Jackson was originally provided to us by the AOTF. It has since gone through some revisions, for which I must take responsibility. The earlier edition that the panel participants had may differ slightly from the version you see here. Panel members have been encouraged to identify where they perceive a fundamental difference between the case they considered and the case that is before you. The case is approximately the same. The four questions, which we will go through in turn, appear at the bottom of the case. We will address question number one first, beginning with Dr. Schultz.

Initial Assessment

Question 1. Based upon your theoretical reference, how do you begin to understand this person? How do you assess and evaluate or understand function/dysfunction?

Sally Schultz
Occupational
Adaptation

I am going to quickly discuss how I understand the individual, how I would assess this individual, and how I would then articulate my perspective on function and dysfunction. Looking at the case that you have, I saw some conflicting elements. However, I do understand that, as an individual in occupational adaptation terms, the patient is "stuck," or *hyperstablized,* in an adaptive response pattern that continually reinforces the state of *occupational dysadaptation.* In other words, her adaptive mechanisms are so impoverished that she really has only one adaptive response from which to draw. The stressors that she experienced, I would expect, exceeded her adaptive capacity. I see an indication that her reservoir of adaptiveness may have, in fact, been somewhat minimal before she experienced these multiple stressors.

To some degree, I would suggest that her career choice, as an administrative clerk, is also indicative of someone who has a need for predictability and imposed order so that she is not required to use her own adaptiveness for successful performance. The multiple stressors overloaded her adaptive capacity and her available mechanisms, that is, her adaptive response.

In terms of assessment, the formulation that I have provided serves as the foundation for this adaptive process. I would want additional information about Dee's past performance and adaptive responses. It would be especially helpful to look at the "goodness-of-fit" between her current adaptive response and previous adaptive responses when she has been faced with significant occupational challenges. She may, in fact, have been predisposed, according to the content of this case, to limited capacity for adaptation. I would suggest that an underlying thinking disorder appears to have come to the surface secondary to the multiple stressors that she experienced. The presence, of course, of the long-standing but guarded thinking disorder will be significant in the course of treatment. The more pervasive this long-standing thinking disorder is, the greater the patient's limitation in becoming more adaptive.

Because Dee is severely decompensated, it is critical to assess in naturalistic settings. Her adaptive response mechanism appears to be basically the same in most experiences of occupational challenge. I would want to see what her range of adaptive response is. To do this, I would observe her and would interact (through occupation rather than words) with her in typical settings, such as during outings, recreation, group time, or leisure activities. Also, the confusion that is indicated in the case study merits, in my opinion, an assessment of her basic cognitive skills. Assessing her psychosocial skills also would be relevant.

Both skill areas (cognitive and psychosocial) could be assessed using a variety of standardized instruments or approaches. However, again, I would include a naturalistic interpretation of her functional skills. Many patients with mental illness can perform in controlled testing situations but fail to function in an occupation-based situation.

Finally, I would want to assess Dee's awareness of her own adaptive response patterns. This assessment would give me an indication, at least initially, of how available she is in terms of learning about the process of occupational adaptation and using that knowledge to influence her own ability to improve relative mastery. Her perception of relative mastery is so low that she has basically abandoned all roles other than being a patient in the hospital.

In terms of function and dysfunction, occupational adaptation views function as the ability to draw sufficiently from a range of adaptive responses to meet the individual's need for relative mastery. Dee's performance would be characterized as dysfunctional in that her choice of adaptive response (a) interferes with her experience of relative mastery in performing her roles, (b) results in unacceptable performance within her occupational environment and respective roles, and (c) perpetuates the state of occupational dysadaptation.

Impairment in her component systems may also be contributing to her dysfunction, in that such impairment impinges on the individual's ability to generate adaptive responses that can lead to a satisfactory level of relative mastery.

Gary Kielhofner
Model of Human Occupation

The approach to the case of Dee was developed in consultation with a number of colleagues. Kathy Baron, Dr. David Baron, Captain Steve Gerardi, Dr. Alexis Henry, and Betty Harland gave input and feedback to my approach to this case.

I must begin by discussing how we use theory. We refer to this process as gathering and reasoning with data. The first step was to use the model as a framework for approaching the initial data of this case and for generating a set of conceptual questions that would guide our data-gathering process. These questions and the information we gathered ultimately led to developing a specific theory of Dee's situation. Hence, we moved from the generic theory that the model presents to the construction of a case-specific theory. More important, this case-specific theory emanated from a dialogue between (a) Dee's point of view and her situatedness in particular circumstances, and (b) a general set of theoretical arguments that provide a way of seeing and explaining.

Gary Kielhofner

By examining the data from the case, we generated the conceptual questions that I will discuss next.

1. In the area of personal causation, a number of circumstances indicate that Dee has extreme loss of control. We would ask questions about what her thoughts and feelings are about control. What parts of her life are most out of control? Conversely, are there any elements that still demonstrate control? What is her sense of control particularly as it relates to substance abuse? I based my approach on the first version of this case, which differs in some regards from the version contained in the handouts today. The later version indicates that Dee was diagnosed as having abused alcohol and it refers to a longstanding maladaptive pattern. Using those case materials, I concluded that Dee's substance abuse was not secondary to her trauma in Saudi Arabia, but instead was part of a long-standing, maladaptive pattern of substance abuse. The materials do not contain enough data to confirm this conclusion, but to go forward with the case, I had to draw some working assumptions.

I would ask Dee what her beliefs are about her abilities. Has she had a history of deficit performance over time? I am assuming that this problem may well be the case. One of the cues to this problem is the comment in the first version of the case that suggested Dee had a long-standing maladaptive pattern. Another cue is that her military rank is lower than it should be, given 11 years of performance; this suggests that she has either been demoted or passed over for promotion. Once again, I am assuming that her rank of only E-5 may be related to chronic substance abuse.

2. In the area of values, I would ask questions about her particular view of life, of her career, and of motherhood. What relative value does she attach to work, to family, and to other aspects of her life? What major values have been disrupted, and in what way does she view them as having been disrupted by current events? How does she view herself in the context of those values? Also, I would want to know what major cultural, religious, or other influences are in Dee's system of values. I would try to get at answers more from her point of view

3. In the area of interests, I would ask the following: What aspects of her life are most satisfying? What aspects of parenting or clerking are satisfying? What was the specific job she did in the military? What did she find most satisfying or dissatisfying? What other interests characterize her lifestyle? And finally, because of my assumptions about her substance abuse, I would ask these questions: Has she been replacing satisfaction and plea-

sure in activity with substance abuse (which is a common pattern)? If so, for how long?

4. In terms of the volitional narrative, I would ask: What has been this woman's main life story, and where does she see her future headed? Why is she uncommitted, or only marginally committed, to occupational therapy as indicated in the case? Was her lack of commitment, for example, related to negative environmental incentives for recovery, which I think may be an issue in this case, or was it related to her perception of the relevance of occupational therapy activities to her volitional narrative?

5. These questions would deal with roles: What value does she attach to various roles, and what are her expectations for filling roles in the future?

6. These questions would deal with habits: What was her habit pattern like before this recent set of events? What impact, if any, did substance abuse have on that habit pattern? What were the most adaptive and maladaptive aspects of her routine?

7. I would ask these questions in terms of the mind-brain-body performance subsystem: What is her skill level at present? My assumption, based on the data given in the case, is that she did not have a long-standing, major skill deficit.

8. In terms of her environment, I would like to know something about the kind of living situation she might be able to return to. What family, neighborhood, and cultural environment conditions she might face?

9. Another area to focus on is her life history pattern. Organization of a human system is the function of the ongoing pattern of action. I want to know what her pretraumatic lifestyle pattern was. What were the adaptive and maladaptive elements? What is the current trajectory of thought and feeling in her behavior? Within this area, I would focus particularly on her experience in therapy to date.

Our research into the meaning of therapy suggests that we should strongly consider how Dee views therapy (Helfrich & Kielhofner, 1994). To be effective, therapy must become an event within the patient's life story, and the fact that Dee is not motivated to participate in activities suggests that therapy has not effectively integrated itself into the stream of her life. Unless her participation in therapy begins to address, at both a feeling and practical level, some opportunity for control over the things she cares about, it is not likely to be effective.

Finally, the following are data-gathering instruments that I would use in her treatment. I will discuss them further when addressing

Gary Kielhofner   how I would go about her therapy. You can refer to the handouts
for descriptions of these assessments and related references (See
Appendix B: Model of Human Occupation). The assessments I selected to answer the above questions about Dee were developed by
using the model of human occupation. All of these assessments
have been subjected to empirical studies to determine and improve
reliability and validity. If time and resources for treatment are
limited, many of the assessments can be integrated into treatment groups.

First, I would use the Occupational Performance History Interview (OPHI), an interview developed for use with the model (see
Appendix B). One reason that I would use the OPHI is that it is a
historical interview and I want to know something about her history. Another reason for my confidence in this instrument is that
the OPHI has a substantial history of being used in research. For
instance, a study completed recently by Henry, Tohen, Coster, and
Tickle-Degnen (1994) found the OPHI valuable in predicting postdischarge outcomes for people who are hospitalized with psychiatric
problems. The OPHI would provide data on values, personal causation, interests, roles, habits, and the environment. While the OPHI
was not originally developed with the concept of volitional narrative in mind, we have done research on the character of narrative
data obtained from the OPHI (Mallinson, Kielhofner, & Mattingly,
1996) and have developed guidelines for gathering and analyzing
narrative data from the OPHI (Mallinson & Kielhofner, 1995).

I would use the Role Checklist (1988) to assess how Dee saw
her past, present, and future roles, and to ascertain what value she
placed on her occupational roles (see Appendix B). The Role
Checklist is generally easy for patients to complete. For depressed
patients, in particular, it can be useful in helping them to recognize
and affirm past role performance. Since Dee has been able to maintain several occupational roles in the past, the instrument should
provide her some opportunity both to reflect on this background
and to begin to anticipate roles in the future.

I would use the Occupational Questionnaire (1986), which has
a substance abuse version that would give information about her
habit pattern, the volitional quality of her occupational performance, and the relationship of substance abuse to her habit pattern.
I would use neither the formal Assessment of Motor and Process
Skills or AMPS (Fisher, 1994) nor the Assessment of Communication and Interaction Skills or ACIS (Forsyth, Salamy, Simon, &
Kielhofner, 1995), because I do not think that Dee has a permanent
skill deficit. I do suspect she has a temporary problem of depressed
process skills and a problem of communication interaction skills.

I would monitor her through informal evaluations and, only if indicated by such screening, I would consider formal use of the AMPS or ACIS.

Last, I would use the Self-Assessment of Occupational Functioning or SAOF (Baron & Curtin, 1990). The twofold value of this assessment is that it would give information about how Dee sees herself. Moreover, the SAOF is organized to arrive at a mutual, goal-setting process. I would like to mention that Henry et al. (1994), in the study mentioned before, found the SAOF to be predictive of postdischarge functioning.

Florence Clark
Occupational Science

How do we begin to understand Dee, given the key concepts listed in Appendix C: Occupational Science, Table 4? I will begin by Addressing the notion of "resistance to the medical model and disciplinary practices." First, in looking at this case, we realized that we were given the institutional narrative only, not Dee's narrative. The institution is controlling the narrative—it's controlling Dee's life at this time. Decisions are made about where she is going to be moved, about what ward she is going to, and about whether or not she will be discharged from the military. We do not get the sense that Dee is participating in her own situation at all. In fact, when Dee does try to assume a bit of control, when at one point she wants to talk about Saudi Arabia in an interview, the therapist complains that Dee would not focus on her future (meet the therapist's expectation) and would talk only about Saudi Arabia (following her own inclination). Dee is not conforming to the social expectations of the power structure; when she attempts to take control of the conversation, her act is interpreted as inappropriate.

Second, medical practitioners are controlling the unfolding of Dee's life. The institution is controlling the decision making. For example, even when Dee's taking of medication is described, what is conveyed is a power discourse. The case description states that "Dee was placed on medication," not that she agreed to take antidepressant drugs. The entire narrative is written in a way that appropriates control, gives it to the power structure, and subjugates the person. To our group, the military hospital seems to be an environment replete with disciplinary practices. Dee is categorized, is classified, and has no voice in this case. In the case description we do not hear Dee's voice in even one paragraph.

We noted that disciplinary practices were used in an attempt to normalize Dee. For example, the first thing we learn about her is age (33 years old), marital status (separated), and gender (female), Then we learn about her psychiatric diagnosis, her occupational classification, and her work status classification. We are given classification

Florence Clark

after classification of a human being. She was punished, restricted, and confined when she failed to conform to expectations, and she continued to be included in groups that it seemed apparent she did not want to attend. Eventually, she was confined physically to spaces (a locked ward) where she was forced to participate in occupational therapy (OT). Our group perceived her as a subjugated individual who was being manipulated in an environment that is actually controlling her narrative and in which she has no voice.

To move on to the second key construct, we embraced the position that to develop a comprehensive view of Dee, we would need to consider the notion that different selves are constructed through occupation in the context of one's life. We assumed that Dee's personhood is distributed across the settings in which she engages in multiple selves. To understand the many facets of Dee, our group stressed that we would need to acquire a sense of the cultures in which she has existed—the army, civilian hospital, military hospital, home, and so forth. We would carefully appraise those cultures, their normative expectations, and the match or mismatch relative to Dee's needs. Our sense was that at the moment Dee is not in the process of self-construction. We would understand her, rather, as in the process of self-deconstruction. However, our reading of Kondo (1990) suggested that Dee's self has the capacity to remold itself in shifting contexts of power and meaning. We would need to understand the connection between Dee's Saudi Arabia experience and the self she is now experiencing, her history in the army, and even her childhood occupations.

Third, our group believed that to understand Dee, we would need to understand her system of meaning. Dee's narrative interpretation of herself as an occupational being would have to be the centerpiece of treatment. We would need to get a sense of what has happened to Dee in Dee's terms. The themes for therapeutic intervention identified by the therapist must be scrutinized, questioned, and even possibly rejected. For example, the idea of occupational role disruption might be an oversimplistic interpretation of what is really going on. Given her history of maladaptive behavior, we have to ask about the context of this behavior and why this case was so vague about what the behavior was. Why were we led to believe that she might, for example, have an alcohol abuse problem? If she did, why was this not overtly stated in the case I received? The confusing elements and vagueness of the case maximized the possibility of misconceptions about Dee. It simply is not clear whether Dee has had a history of substance abuse. Further, it is unclear why we should be concerned about her inability to formulate future issues or why the clinician seemed unconcerned about what was on

Dee's mind at the time the case was written. Why did the therapist interpret Dee's inability to focus on the future as a problem? It was unclear why the future was the therapist's preeminent concern.

Our group thought that in the interview process, Dee should be encouraged to talk about Saudi Arabia since we were given clues that this experience was on her mind and was what she wanted to discuss. Through the interview process, we thought the therapist should attempt to get an idea of how Dee is making sense of her life, what she is using to organize her experiences, what she wishes to gain in her future, how past events are affecting her current understanding of life, where she is in the story of herself as an occupational being at this moment, and why after so many years she is now questioning army life. Why now?

Next, in seeking to gain a sense of Dee, we would turn to the idea that meaningful occupation has powerful transformative potential. To identify the occupations with the greatest therapeutic valence, we reasoned that we would have to understand the impact of the contexts in which Dee has been—Saudi Arabia, the medical hospital, the army hospital, civilian hospital, her home life. We would have to identify meaningful themes that could interest Dee in occupation. We extracted from the case description that Saudi Arabia, her children, and service are possible meaningful themes. I must remind you that the version of the case I received stated that Dee was interested in doing things for children and in doing service. That statement is not in the version you were given today. The revised sentence would substantially change our whole approach to intervention.

To gain a sense of the occupational contexts that had therapeutic potential, we needed to generate hypotheses about Dee's responsiveness to normative practices. Our group gained a sense from the case that Dee was not responsive to group intervention and at the moment does not want to return to work. She apparently doesn't want to be or is not ready to be normalized. She doesn't seem to want to conform, nor does she seem to be compelled to fit into the prevailing military culture. We conceived one approach to intervention: examine the ways of not fitting in and still having a happy life. We imagined that it might be possible for Dee to build a life that would satisfy her and that would not depend on social conformity. Using Lave's (1988) description of cognition in practice, we reasoned that Dee's poor work performance and poor focus on work may be exacerbated by the situation in which she finds herself— that is, in a military hospital. If she were in another context, Lave's work suggests she might be better able to perform.

Finally, we would have to understand Dee as the protagonist in her own social drama. A breach has occurred in her life. Her

Florence Clark
husband's abandonment and betrayal, his spending of the family savings, the abandonment of her children, and the Saudi Arabia experience all create a breach or a break in her own narrative of who she is as an occupational being. The crisis seems to have resulted in withdrawal and depression, and now she appears to be in a regressive phase in which she is hospitalized. According to Turner's (1987) theory, this may be a time for stock-taking and self-scrutinizing. This phase can result in irrevocable schism, reintegration, or reorganization. It appears that Dee will return to civilian life, so our understanding is that what is of primary importance is to assist her in doing that successfully.

Appendix C: Occupational Science, Table 6, lists the Assessment Strategy. Assessment would be based on hermeneutic interview techniques and observations of Dee in all of the contexts in which she finds herself. The assessment would be ongoing and processual, and through it an understanding of Dee as an occupational being with situationally specific identities and capabilities would emerge. Framing Dee's case in terms of function and dysfunction may lead to reductionism that would create a disempowering context for Dee and may lead to a mechanized form of intervention. What Dee needs to do is begin the process of self-reconstruction. She needs to be given the time and space to figure out strategies for dealing with the breach in the social drama she is experiencing, for dealing with this crisis, for piecing together an emerging identity through engagement in meaningful occupation, and for creating herself as an occupational being in the future.

Intervention Process

Question 2. Based upon your theoretical reference, how would you begin the intervention process? Or, how would factors influencing the unfolding of the person's story be considered?

Sally Schultz
Occupational
Adaptation
My comments will be based on what I would do from an occupational adaptation perspective in the initial stage of therapy. Intervention would, of course, be based on the results of the assessment. I will proceed with my comments about the intervention method from the formulation that I provided you earlier, which in essence says that I am operating under the assumption that Dee has a long-standing, impoverished repertoire of adaptive response. Her need for predictability within the occupational environment is significant, and her need to limit the demand on her adaptive response mechanism is also significant. Because of the severity of her present state, I will focus therapy on helping her regain or obtain ad-

ditional adaptive responses that are positive rather than focusing on future directions. Treatment will focus on the immediate, the here, and the now. This focus will be accomplished readily through concrete occupational activities that are not closely related to her role of mother or worker.

Her response shows that the occupational challenges embedded within those two roles now exceed and overpower her present adaptive capacity. I would reframe the therapy described in the case study in a way that allows her to engage in a variety of media. Because of the severity of Dee's current status, the therapist will have to initially determine which occupations the patient may find most therapeutic. Of course, that determination can be facilitated by comments and critique from Dee insofar as she is capable of contributing at this time.

The occupations that would be the most therapeutic are those in which the inherent challenge does not exceed the adaptive responses that Dee has available and that would allow her to experience a sufficient level of relative mastery. Though she may, in fact, need occupational readiness—learning coping strategies, relaxation techniques, social skills, substance abuse education, and so forth—I think that at this point (the beginning of the therapy process), such skill-based learning should be delayed until Dee has a more positive orientation toward her ability to influence her environment and has a sense of relative mastery.

I would postpone those groups that are discharge-oriented or future-focused. The more such groups are imposed on the patient (i.e., not meaningful), the more extreme will be her reluctance to participate or gain any benefit from them. In fact, from an occupational adaptation frame of reference, I would not see her behavior as manipulative in a negative sense. I would, in fact, see her behavior as attempts to avoid the groups that are inappropriate for her, rather than seeing her as being inappropriate for the group. Dee's response indicates that either she is being overwhelmed by the group or she simply does not value the experiences there. In either case, the group is therapeutically counterproductive.

As Dee experiences increased relative mastery within occupations in which she feels safe enough to engage, the therapist's task will be one of progressively grading the occupational challenge that the particular occupation offers. Such grading of the occupational challenge must occur naturalistically. As the challenge increases, the demand for adaptive response will show a consonant increase. Dee will then be ready to begin assimilating new skills that are relevant to adaptive responses and that are called for within the context of the roles she has abandoned.

Gary Kielhofner
Model of Human
Occupation

I will propose a possible sequence of intervention in the next section as I am speaking about anticipated outcomes. In this section, I will provide a rationale and considerations for Dee's treatment using a conceptualization of her occupational function and dysfunction while focusing on the interrelationship of volition, habituation, and environmental influences.

Volitional structure is generated and sustained by experience. We can certainly observe now that Dee's volition includes maladaptive elements, but what is more important, we must recognize the underlying experiences that have generated this maladaptive volition. Recognizing these experiences will help us to think about what new experiences might enable Dee to reorganize her volition.

Dee seems to value work and parenting. The loss of her job and the disruption of her caretaker role with her children have likely generated feelings of loss of worth, along with a heightened sense of helplessness and depression. Moreover, Dee's personal causation was likely vulnerable premorbidly as a result of what appears to be marginal performance in the military associated with substance abuse. In addition, her loss of financial resources (i.e., her husband having squandered their life savings) most likely exacerbated her feeling out of control. Dee is a middle-class individual in a society that lacks the extensive social and economic supports for the middle class that are present, for example, in Swedish society. Consequently, middle-class people who meet financial difficulty in the United States can face catastrophic results. This potential catastrophe, in turn, can create a tremendous sense of being out of control.

Finally, I think it is quite possible that Dee has fallen into a negative and desperate coping style for getting control. After all, her symptomatology and her inability to function have resulted in a positive financial incentive, namely, a military discharge with disability. I am not saying that she is actively manipulating circumstances to this end. Nonetheless, the reality is that Dee has gotten secondary gain from her sustained illness, at a time when these economic consequences are very consequential to her and her children.

Other evidence that supports my conclusion is her symptom cluster. I shared the case with a psychiatrist-diagnostician who felt that the symptoms did not fit together in a syndromatic pattern. This analysis suggests that Dee's ongoing symptomatology and her difficulty engaging in therapy are strongly influenced by current environmental circumstances and incentives. In a sense, we should not be entirely surprised at Dee's condition, because her environment is not currently pressing for and affording more adaptive occupational behavior.

We have very little information relating to her interests, but when Dee does get to the point of reestablishing her lifestyle, consideration of interests will be very important to help her create and sustain a satisfying pattern of occupation.

In terms of Dee's volitional narrative, I would proceed on the following logic. Our research on narratives suggests that we have to consider how Dee has narrated her life. In interpreting Dee's volitional narrative, we could use an approach we developed (Mallinson & Kielhofner, 1996); this approach involves understanding the underlying metaphor in her personal narrative. I expect that entrapment (one of the metaphors we identified in the volitional narratives of people hospitalized for psychiatric illness) is the likely metaphor that drives her narrative. In our study (Mallinson & Kielhofner, 1996), we found that this type of narrative is associated with many features of Dee's case, including depression and suicidal idealization. Entrapment narratives are powerful and can paralyze volitional outlook and decisions. Understanding Dee's volitional narrative as such gives us a way to begin to organize therapy as a relevant set of events within her larger story.

I would somewhat disagree with Sally's approach to Dee; our research (Helfrich & Kielhofner, 1994) indicates that patients see all activities (whether or not those activities are designed to be relevant to the personal narrative) from the perspective of their volitional narratives and interpreted in terms of it. I think it is unavoidable that the occupations we use in therapy will be experienced by patients in relationship to their own lives. Patients do not come into therapy; therapy comes into patients' lives.

If I ascertained that Dee's volitional structure is dominated by a sense of being trapped, my therapy would be to organize therapeutic events as strategies for getting her out of the trap. I believe this approach is most likely to have success. Such an approach also requires that we examine the narrative's correspondence to Dee's real-life situations. One may express concern about the oppressiveness of roles, but the reality is that this is a woman who has two children, who lives in a real world, and who has real expectations. To change her narrative, she will have to change the circumstances of her life, so an interaction must exist between the telling and the behaving of the volitional narrative.

Habituation is an internalization of ways of traversing our habitats. It's no small matter that Dee has been, in recent months, displaced to another part of the globe and has been, through her hospitalization, separated from normal work and living environments. Habituation is maintained by the repetition of patterns of

Gary Kielhofner

behavior and by one's familiar temporal and social habitats. It is also important to consider how patterns of behavior have been disrupted and can be reinstated for Dee. Until recently, she maintained worker and caretaker roles. The length of time one is removed from roles is correlated negatively with the success in reestablishing roles. For that reason, it would be important to begin immediately, in small increments, to reinstate Dee's role behaviors. Of course, this approach would depend on what relative value she places on roles and on what anticipation she has for future roles along with what will be expected of her by her social environment.

It is important to ensure that occupational forms that were part of her prior roles are used in therapy. For instance, we should not assume that making craft gifts for her children (which, for example, may have been what she was encouraged to do in previous occupational therapy) is an appropriate occupational form to use in therapy. It may be, but her occupational therapy would depend on whether making things for her children was part of her past role script. Such things as making decisions that affect her children's lives, financially planning for them (which seems to be a huge issue for her now), or even reviewing school performance and helping with homework may be more appropriate. Dee should be given the opportunity to access such occupational forms, and the environmental press (i.e., the supports and expectations) should be calibrated to what she is capable of doing.

A similar approach could be taken to Dee's worker role, but I am assuming her immediate priority would be her maternal role.

Scaffa's (1991) research suggests that erosion of work habits is a likely consequence of alcoholism. Johnson's (1995) research also suggests that leisure time becomes dominated by alcohol abuse, and I would expect that, to an extent, both Dee's work and leisure habits have been eroded. Hence, we need to pay attention to the reorganization of her habit structure.

In summary, I think it is important to recognize how volition, habituation, and environmental factors are together affecting Dee's performance. No single factor can account for her current situation; it is, instead, the whole dynamic situation that accounts for her current occupational dysfunction.

Florence Clark
Occupational Science

I am puzzled as to why, if Dee has had a history of alcohol abuse, that piece of information wasn't stated explicitly in the case. I think that Gary's piecing together really makes a lot of sense, but I am curious as to why the alcohol abuse wasn't stated since it seems to be a crucial factor if it is part of Dee's picture. I will now address the factors to be considered from the perspective I have been offering today and on the basis of the version of the case I received. The factors are listed in Appendix C: Occupational Science, Table 7. Earlier, I stated that we were given the institutional narrative on Dee and that we must examine it in terms of disciplinary practices, which I have done in my interpretation.

Because we have no information about Dee from her own perspective or in her own "voice," our only option is to excavate this vague institutional narrative to detect clues about who Dee is as an occupational being. What themes might inspire Dee to engage in transformative occupation? How is she oriented in relation to past, present, and future? How does she perceive her current situation and its resolution in terms of social drama? What is interfering with her progress? Why isn't she responsive to occupational therapy? These are some of the factors that we must consider. What were her childhood occupations? This information is not provided in the institutional narrative, so we must try to retrieve it from the assessment process. How does Dee conceive of motherhood? What was her history in high school and what were her post-army experiences? Were they positive, negative, or mixed? What were her motives for joining the army? We have to understand Dee's intentionality. It is important to know if Dee's husband is still in her life. How are the children doing? Is Dee's mother able to care for them? What is Dee's civilian life going to consist of (employment, home, support systems)? We need to piece together a picture of what kind of future Dee might have, even if she does not have it right now. It might be good for the therapist to have some sense of her future. How can Dee's vision for herself be realized through occupation?

I will now discuss how we would begin the intervention process. I have summarized our approach to the intervention process in Appendix C: Occupational Science, Table 8. First, we would place the narrative in Dee's control and strive for patient-centered rather than institution-centered care. Dee would author the story of herself as an occupational being in the future. She and her therapist would collaborate in enacting a story that would unfold as Dee's future. I call this process occupational story making (making a future, building a future, and making decisions). Dee's narrative of herself as an occupational being would be rebuilt by connecting elements of her past self with her emerging self. She would define the problems to be worked on through engaging in an occupation. What are the issues or the threats right now that she perceives need to be worked on? What does she want to work on? The focus would

Florence Clark   probably be on the present and the immediate past. I agree with
                        Dr. Schultz's earlier statements on present issue. The therapist
                        would assist Dee in resolving the social drama that has become
                        Dee's life. We would look at the reorganization of her new civilian
                        life as a primary issue.

                        One of my students, Brenda Scroggins, said that "Occupations
                        are not put in our life; they are out of our lives." Thus we excavated
                        this case to figure out what sort of projects Dee would be interested
                        in doing right now. I agree with Dr. Schultz here too; Dee is moti-
                        vated to work on projects directed toward service to others and her
                        children. Right now, this service is what she can handle. Because
                        the version of the case I received stated that Dee was interested in
                        service and projects with her children, our group found this state-
                        ment to be a crucial clue as to where to begin therapy.

                        An important consideration in Dee's intervention is how to safely
                        return Dee to her family context—if that return is what she wants.
                        If she is suicidal, what must be done to ensure that she returns
                        safely? Is she an alcoholic? We must consider these issues. We
                        would use extra structural settings and times in the early stages of
                        intervention. The intervention would be highly unregimented, in-
                        dividualized, and without pressure to conform so we could resist
                        duplicating the normative and disciplinary practices that Dee seems
                        to be rejecting.

                        We would give Dee the time to work through the frustration and
                        confusion she had experienced in Saudi Arabia—just give her time.
                        Concerns about the future can be addressed later in the therapeutic
                        process. We would assist Dee in identifying and engaging in occu-
                        pations that might help her resolve her situation and move forward
                        in the story of herself as an occupational being. Renee McDannel,
                        one of the doctoral students, suggested that we might encourage
                        Dee to give parties for her own and other children or to do crafts
                        for them if that interests her. Other options for tapping into Dee's
                        interest in service to others might include preparing dining experi-
                        ences for other people or orchestrating celebrations, thereby build-
                        ing on the hint in the case description that Dee likes to do things
                        for her children and for others. We would stimulate her to envision
                        herself as a civilian. Ms. McDannel suggested this vision might
                        occur by having her search magazines about civilian life. To help
                        Dee work through feelings about her Saudi Arabia experience and
                        to resolve any issues that she is finding disturbing, we might en-
                        courage her to create an art book on the meaning of those emotions.
                        Working on seemingly mundane activities that address her current
                        concerns might help. She should also be encouraged to deal with

phone calls, pay bills, and do household tasks. In this area I agree with Dr. Kielhofner; ritual might be used to resolve the breaches in her narrative.

Intervention Outcomes

Question 3. Based upon your theoretical reference, what are projected outcomes for this person?

Sally Schultz
Occupational
Adaptation

I do not propose that the patient's future or past is irrelevant. However, given what I read in the case, I would be concerned that Dee's ability to report a valid narrative is compromised at this time. Just as I would not focus initial therapy on the future, I would want to diminish the significance of the past, until a sufficient level of relative mastery is obtained, so that the narrative that I based treatment on would be more rich.

In terms of outcomes, the occupational adaptation frame of reference specifically defines outcomes of intervention. Because the target of therapy is directed at improving the internal adaptation process, I would expect to see some very specific things happening if my treatment approach were working.

1. I would begin to see Dee acquire new or modified adaptive responses.

2. I would begin to see her generalize the changes in her adaptive response repertoire to similar situations with similar demands.

3. I would see her begin to generate positive adaptive responses in novel situations and to novel demands.

4. I would begin to see an increase in the three aspects of relative mastery:

   ■ an improvement in her perception of the efficiency of her occupational performance

   ■ an increase in her perception of her effectiveness in doing these occupations

   ■ an increased satisfaction that she herself experiences and a perception of increased satisfaction to others.

These performance outcomes would lead to a reacquisition of some of her roles and an increased acceptance of future orientation. At this point the significance of the past and the future becomes integrated into the therapy process. Until such a time, Dee's ability to benefit from the necessary readiness training and to accept the occupational challenges congruent with her mother and worker role could exceed her adaptive capacity.

Sally Schultz

The outcome of therapy is oriented at changes in the adaptive response mechanisms. I have outlined how those changes are evidenced and how we can actually observe those changes. Even though adaptation is an internal process, we can observe that adaptation is happening. When adaptation begins, the past and the future can become tools to help Dee be more adaptive in those occupational environments and in roles that have been lost.

Gary Kielhofner
Model of Human Occupation

My first comments will not be what I was prepared to say, but instead come from thinking about what the other two presenters have just argued. I hadn't planned to mention this, but I now feel it is relevant to examine Dee's Saudi Arabia experience and her diagnosis of posttraumatic stress syndrome.

Military literature indicates that posttraumatic stress syndrome was extremely rare in the Desert Storm experience. In particular, it was almost nonexistent in noncombat troops, of which Dee was a part. Dee, almost assuredly, never witnessed any conflict. So we have to ask ourselves these questions: What was the trauma? What was the stress that she faced?

Betty Harlan, who gave me input on the case from the perspective of her own military experience, suggested the following thesis. It appears that Dee's trauma is much more related to separation from her home and small children, followed by her return home to learn that her husband had left, had given her children to her mother, and had depleted their financial resources. The trauma is not the Saudi Arabia experience, but the deprivation it created and the shock she faced upon her return.

I suspect Dee is focused on Saudi Arabia because, while she is extremely dysfunctional now, 3 months ago she was a soldier, functioning as a clerk and doing well enough to be deployed internationally. I believe that she is focusing on Saudi Arabia not because it was traumatic, but because it was the last experience she has to hold onto in which she was functioning adequately in a role. I think she is struggling to hold onto something that validates her as a competent being and, therefore, that has meaning for her. It is precisely for this reason that I think it is important to move her to the future where she can find validation. I am confident that one could obtain from Dee a sufficient narrative to appreciate how she is seeing the world and to begin to work toward a future narrative.

The actual sequence of Dee's treatment would depend on several factors, including her mood, her functional level, her resources and constraints in the treatment setting, and so forth. My assumptions concerning these factors are largely implicit in what I will propose. However the assessment is organized, I would like to integrate assessment into the course of treatment and to collect data along the way.

I think that Dee is clearly not in control of her life or her treatment, and I would first want to put her in control of her treatment. To do this, I would begin with the SAOF (Kielhofner, 1995). My aim would be to facilitate Dee's first steps in defining her own situation and her first steps in getting control of treatment as she determines what her first simple treatment goal would be.

I would firmly and supportively point out to Dee that she is very likely to feel less depressed if she begins to move toward doing something that is important to her. Our experience with the SAOF is that it is extremely useful for patients who have been labeled as resistive. I think that Florence is correct in rejecting the label of Dee as a resistive person and that we need to see Dee as a person who is responding negatively to therapy that has not met her needs. Patients who feel hopeless must see therapy as helpful and relevant to their life narrative to be able to derive a sense of hope about the future.

At this point in intervention, I would also make informal observations (as Sally suggested) of Dee's skill level. I would use as a framework for observation the concepts of *process* and *communication and interaction* skills. Because I expect any skill deficits to be temporary, I would focus on appropriate adaptations in activities to minimize the disruption in Dee's carrying out activities to achieve her goals. Minimizing disruptions would ensure that Dee does not become unnecessarily frustrated or discouraged.

I would ask Dee, as she is able, to complete the Role Checklist (Kielhofner, 1995). As I noted earlier, patients often find identifying their past roles a very affirming process, and in the context of acknowledging their past functioning, they are able to aim for roles in the future. I would administer and discuss the Role Checklist with Dee, to get at her valued roles and at the activities related to those roles; I would expect Dee to identify parent and worker as her valued roles.

On the way back to reclaiming her roles and reestablishing her habits, Dee is very likely to be affected by the volitional narrative of entrapment. She may feel extremely overwhelmed by the responsibilities of becoming a single parent (a likely scenario for her in the future). She may worry about how her children will view her after her current illness and hospitalization and how they will accept mothering from her. She may feel unqualified and anxious about a civilian job. Addressing all these issues, step by step, will be necessary to build up her future volitional narrative. At the same time as we reinstate Dee's roles and habits, I would move her

Gary Kielhofner

toward identifying new short-term goals with specific activities to be pursued both inside and outside occupational therapy.

I would use the Occupational Questionnaire to see how Dee has spent her time in the past and how she currently spends her time. I would focus on how Dee could adaptively structure her time through the week and build activities related to her roles into her routine. I would address incorporating leisure interests, which can foster a satisfying lifestyle.

Through this process, I would learn more about Dee's volitional narrative and incremental pieces and would assist her in shaping a positive volitional narrative for the future. At an appropriate time, but probably not immediately, I would conduct the Occupational Performance History Interview (Kielhofner, 1995) to get a more detailed occupational history.

I expect that at different points in therapy Dee is going to become overwhelmed and perhaps resistant to some of my suggestions. At such times, a very calculated approach to volition is needed, an approach that builds on her life story—a life story envisioned by the therapist and the patient together. An alliance of the patient and the therapist to pursue this volitional narrative would be important to the therapist's ability to nudge her along.

The volitional story is not simply told or anticipated; it must be enacted to sustain its direction and its value as a motivational force in Dee's life. Recent research in our department by Trudy Mallinson has examined the latent-trait structure of the occupational performance history interviews from two different psychiatric data sets. In both cases, the findings point to the fact that patients face a larger challenge in enacting than in telling their volitional narratives. Following through on role behavior and maintaining habit structure is more difficult than formulating a volitional narrative. Therapy to help Dee envision her story in positive ways will be important work. Nonetheless, given her recent circumstances and trauma, a larger challenge will be to actualize these elements in her daily life.

Another important consideration to address in therapy is Dee's environment, in particular Dee's relationship to her mother and to the stability of the grandparent household. Here are some major questions to consider: Will the grandmother support Dee's transition back into the major caretaking role with the children? Will Dee be joining her mother's household when Dee is away from the hospital, is out during day hospitalization, and is finally discharged. A plan for each of these transition phases must be worked out in association with Dee's mother and, if possible, Dee's mother should be brought into a partnership.

Although Dee has a number of serious problems and a major disruption of all her life roles and habit structure, she does appear to have some strengths to build upon. Even if she has had a substance abuse problem of some duration, she has been able to maintain a consistent role as a worker in the military. It also appears that Dee has been able to accomplish things as saving money.

If Dee's marriage ends, as I am assuming it will, and if Dee's mother is emotionally supportive and provides a transitional household wherein Dee can reassume the maternal role, it's possible that Dee can reinstate that role. It is also possible that she can find employment, although whether she can manage both roles simultaneously will have to be carefully considered.

My goals would be to reinstate her maternal and home-maintainer roles (assuming these are also her goals), followed by exploring whether and when to reinstate her worker role. I would certainly try to create affordance and press both in our treatment and in her home and family environment so Dee can resume roles as swiftly as is possible for her. The longer she stays out of roles, the less likely she will be to return successfully to them.

If work becomes a goal in therapy, I would probably conduct a secondary evaluation focused on work. In particular, the Worker Role Interview, or WRI (Velozo, Kielhofner, & Fisher, 1990), and the Work Environment Impact Scale, or WEIS (Velozo, Moore-Corner, & Kielhofner, 1996), may be appropriate to assess Dee's work-related strengths and weaknesses and her work environment needs. The WRI has been found to be predictive of return to work of persons with physical injuries. One study suggests the WRI is a valid assessment for psychiatric populations. The WEIS has been studied with a psychiatric population and appears to be a valid assessment. Both would be helpful in setting treatment goals and in making recommendations to Dee for overseeing her own discharge behavior, beginning a job-search strategy, and getting referrals to vocational services or work training.

Florence Clark
Occupational Science

In his recent book on professionalism, Friedson (1994) states

> The way one conceives of health care tasks and outcomes reflects the way one conceives of the people being treated. Standardizing the conception of tasks and outcomes for purposes of measuring and controlling them also standardizes the conception of people and their difficulties . . . people are reduced to formally defined categories. They become objects produced by reliable methods at a predictable cost. While the bureaucratic method may solve the problem of trust by its reliability, it undermines the flexible, discretionary judgment that is necessary to adapt services to individuals' needs (p. 194).

Florence Clark   What can I say about outcomes when I am given a page and a
quarter of institutionalized categorical jargon describing a patient
whom I have never talked to and whom I do not know at all as an
occupational being? Lave (1988) wrote, "What happens in the real
world is dependent upon intentionality and the obdurate features of
the environment." I cannot predict what is going to happen in this
case because I don't know much about Dee's intentionality, and we
don't know much about the environment to which she will return
in civilian life. We have only a vague sense of those factors from the
case. It would be presumptuous of us, at this point, to think about
outcomes in any kind of specific sense.

More generally, what we need to do is to help Dee make sensitive and reasonably accurate judgments about her potential.
Deborah Mandel, a doctoral student, wrote in her case analysis,
"[We can hope] Dee will come to value her own voice and begin
to see a multitude of futurelike stories for herself as an occupational
being." Dee will come to understand herself as an occupational
being, understand the process by which one crafts oneself through
occupation, be informed about the power and disciplinary structures that are impinging on her life, and resolve the crisis in which
she now finds herself. Penny Richardson accomplished these things
in her case study (Clark, 1993). I would like to see Dee make similar accomplishments. That is the extent to which I can speak about
outcomes.

Future Clinical Research

Question 4. What research questions are viable or needed to study clinical application of your work?

Sally Schultz   I would like to emphasize that from an occupational adaptation
Occupational   perspective, I would engage Dee in the here and now during the
Adaptation   initial part of therapy and provide her with experiences of relative
mastery without the threat of becoming less depressed. My expe-
rience with individuals with severe major depression is that the opportunity to lose the depression is actually experienced by patients
as being thrust into facing occupational challenges that they know
they are incapable of meeting. The following questions outline
broad categories of research needed on occupational adaptation.
The first questions focus on evaluation and assessment.

■ **Research Question 1.** What procedures will best clarify the nature of the client's internal adaptive response process? This
question is a vital area for further research because the internal
adaptive process is a target of therapy. More methods are criti-
cally needed to determine what that process is about.

■ **Research Question 2.** What is the relationship between the different forms of occupational activity and the development of rich adaptive responses across a life span?

■ **Research Question 3.** Is there an identifiable pattern of change that is experienced as a client becomes increasingly adaptive?

■ **Research Question 4.** What type of occupational experiences will lead to acquisition of new internal adaptive responses?

Gary Kielhofner
Model of Human Occupation

Conceptual practice models, such as the model of human occupation, are an especially effective way to organize the development of knowledge and to guide research. Models incorporate theoretical arguments that are interwoven and that provide an explanation of function and dysfunction along with a rationale for intervention. Within these theoretical arguments, we can ask both basic and applied research questions.

Basic research tests the theoretical arguments concerning order and disorder (function and dysfunction). However, because we have a theoretical system in which the arguments about order and disorder are linked to the rationale for intervention, such research is directly useful for practice. Research that informs us about adaptive processes in occupation is useful for understanding states of occupational dysfunction and for understanding how persons cope with illness and disability.

Applied research is that which seeks to validate clinical assessments and to test the effectiveness of the model. This research is very helpful in providing evidence concerning the theoretical arguments. For example, the research that we did in developing the Assessment of Communication and Interaction Skills was critical to developing our conceptualization of skill.

When we consider *occupational function,* the following kinds of research questions arise: How are interests, values, personal causation, roles, and habits developed? How do they contribute to adaptive occupational decision making at different life stages? One example is a study by Hans Jonsson, Lena Borell, and me in Stockholm (Jonsson, Kielhofner & Borell, 1997). We have been examining the volitional process by which older persons anticipate and make decisions about retirement. The first in a series of papers coming from this longitudinal study examines the formation of volitional narratives about retirement. In the next phase, we will examine how these volitional anticipations of retirement affected the actual retirement process.

Another example is a study conducted by Laurie Matusiac (1995) in her master's thesis at the University of Illinois at Chicago. Laurie

Gary Kielhofner   conducted a qualitative study of children in the home so she could examine how volition developed and was expressed in toddlers. This more basic research was a prelude to an applied project in which we are developing a clinical tool for assessing volition in children through observation.

Concerning *occupational dysfunction,* we might ask the following: What happens to interests, values, personal causation, roles, and habits in association with different psychosocial and physical dysfunction? How do problems in volition, habituation, and performance contribute to occupational dysfunction? One set of studies compares adaptive to maladaptive groups to see how volition and habituation differ in the two groups. A second set of studies has examined the correlation between the status of volition and habituation with observed occupational function or dysfunction. One example is a study that was completed by Anne Neville-Jan (Neville-Jan, 1994) and that examined the relationship of personal causation, values, and interests to that of occupational productivity in persons with varying levels of depression.

The most powerful kinds of studies are those that ask whether volition, habituation, and performance variables predict performance. One example of such a study was published by Oakley, Kielhofner, and Barris (1985) that showed that variables selected from the model were excellent predictors of adaptive behavior in persons with psychiatric illness. A more recent study by Henry et al. (1994) examined more long-term prediction. Henry gathered data on psychiatric inpatients by using variables and instruments derived from the model, and she was able to show good prediction of function 6 months postdischarge. Still other examples are studies by Craig Velozo and his students at the University of Illinois at Chicago (UIC), who have been using the model-based Worker Role Interview (Velozo, Kielhofner, & Fisher, 1990) to predict the return to work following injury.

At UIC, we have had a strong emphasis on instrument development and measurement research. As a result we have developed an increasingly wide array of clinical tools that have evidence of reliability and validity. Instrument development is important for two reasons. First, these studies have been helpful in sorting out theoretical constructs, and they can provide good measures for research. Second, these studies produce and refine clinical assessments, and they provide evidence of the usefulness and dependability of these assessments.

Our goal is to develop a wide array of useful assessment for a model that can be selected on the basis of the assessments' relevance and suitability for different kinds of patients and in different circumstances. Many of the assessments we have developed are supported through detailed manuals that are available at cost through the Model of Human Occupation Clearinghouse at UIC.

As practitioners, we need studies that examine the utility of the model in practice and its helpfulness for clinical reasoning. An excellent example is a study by Jaime Muñoz and others (Muñoz, Lawlor, & Kielkhofner, 1993) that examined clinical reasoning of 50 therapists using models of human occupation as a frame of reference on psychiatry. That study was very helpful in identifying the clinical utility of various parts of the model.

We also need studies of the therapeutic process to determine how well the theory explains clinical change or the lack thereof. One example is a study published by Helfrich and Kielhofner (1994) that examined the issue of how clients experience therapy and how their volitional narratives affect the meaning of therapy. Another example is a current AOTF-funded project in which Trudy Mallinson, Laura Barret, and I are examining the process and outcomes of therapy in work. Finally, we need outcomes research to examine the effects of therapy that is based on the model; a few such studies have been published, but much more needs to be done.

In summary, I want to emphasize that I consider it important to organize a program of research under the kind of theoretical and practical umbrella that a model of practice represents. Such research contributes to cumulative science and allows the building up of knowledge on a focused topic. Also, because of the structure of models of practice, different kinds of studies such as those I have just discussed can be more readily interrelated and integrated. Finally, I think the clinical relevance of research done from the framework of a model of practice has more ready application in practice.

Florence Clark
Occupational Science

I will address only the particular research questions that were provoked by this case and not those that are of more general concern in occupational science. My discussion is very specific to this case and the kinds of research questions that seem most relevant to it. The research questions are listed in Appendix C: Occupational Science, Table 9.

The first research question asks, "What is the relationship of narrative to engagement in the therapeutic process?" I would like to systematically study what would actually happen as a consequence of an intervention based on the five theoretical constructs listed in Appendix C: Occupational Science, Table 4. What would actually unfold in Dee's therapeutic process when the personal narrative of this patient was excavated in the way that I described, when she was encouraged to engage in occupations that were identified as

Florence Clark

having transformative potential for her, and when those occupations would seem to be capable of redressing the social drama of her life? I would like to see research encouraged that would provide a thick description of the therapeutic process in detail. This research approach could then be used with other cases. At the end of such research projects we would have a set of cases similar to that described in my Eleanor Clarke Slagle lecture—narrative analyses about people's complete transformations that are based on their discovery of themselves as occupational beings. These narratives or stories tell how the people interpret their lives and how they use occupation to bring about transformation that ultimately resolves the crises in which they find themselves. I would like to see more research of that kind.

The second research question asks, "How can narrative be used as a tool to uncover the occupations of greatest potential therapeutic value to specific patients?" This is an extremely important question. I expect it is possible to create exponential changes in people who engage in certain occupations, but how do we identify which occupations have such power? For example, I think that in Dee's case, the scrapbook project may have had such potential, whether it ultimately told the story of a mother's pain caused by separation from a child or by witnessing war. I think that we tend to minimize the therapeutic potential that is embedded in occupation even though it is relevant to meaning systems of patients. We need research that explains how practitioners can discern the occupations that will provide the greatest therapeutic benefit.

The third research question of relevance asks, "Can this genre of intervention—the kind that I described in Dee's case—actually be implemented in existing treatment settings?" Obviously, this treatment approach challenges prevailing ideas about the nature of mental health practice. It would be interesting to explore whether this approach is feasible, given the current administrative structures it might, to some extent, threaten.

A fourth research question of interest asks, "What is the difference in the quality of recovery, physical or emotional, following occupational therapy using this approach when compared to other models?" We need to examine the different trajectories that we see in patients on the basis of how we work with them and what our basic assumptions are about how to proceed with treatment. It would be fascinating to systematically study what would have unfolded had each of us actively treated Dee, given the diversity in the therapeutic approaches we recommend.

Finally, I believe we need research on the changes required so occupational therapy education can produce therapists who would be comfortable using innovative practice methods that are fluid, improvisational, and less structured. We also need to examine strategies for developing practitioners who can be successful advocates for innovative treatment approaches.

Audience Questions

Audience Participant

One of the things I was most impressed with was that each of these approaches takes time. In the current health care system that occupational therapists are facing, particularly in the inpatient psychiatric setting, time is something that we don't have. This case was a little unusual, since in the military we do have a little more time to do some of the things that people are talking about. So, what thoughts have each of you given to reconciling the conflict between the typical length of stay of 5 to 7 days and these approaches, which are clearly ones that involve more than that amount of time?

Sally Schultz

Contrary to what you might think, I would see an occupation adaptation orientation as being directly suitable for the brevity of stay in that the focus is not on a long progression of skill development but on a progression of adaptive responses that would allow the person to generalize skills more immediately.

Gary Kielhofner

My quick answer is that some aspects of the model have been developed and adapted for short-term settings. Additionally, I would assert that we must be careful to look at changes in the health care structure and not assume that we are victims of those changes. We need to ask, "What role are we taking to organize the health care structure?"

Illinois mental health care has almost completely shifted from inpatient care to community-based care. Jobs in community mental health are not specifically occupational therapy jobs, but occupational therapists can do those jobs. For example, here in Chicago, Cathy Burson, an occupational therapist, is employed by the state of Illinois' mental health system and has worked effectively to convince administrators that they should have a mental health approach based in part on the model of human occupation. She had to know how to package and present the ideas to them and had to sell them on the idea that she had a useful understanding and approach to solving the problems of mental health patients.

Gary Kielhofner   If we do the right kinds of things, we will see new, nontraditional jobs emerge. We must use these theoretical ideas to change the delivery system and not worry about how we will create ideas that will fit into what we think the delivery system will demand of us.

Florence Clark   I agree with Gary. I do want to say that I believe that occupational therapy has become an ally of our grave diggers. We have been developing the technologies that could result in our destruction as a profession, in the sense that the termites of reductionism have so infested our practice that 10 years from now, I am afraid practice will become so simplistic that we will not need humans to do it; rather, computers will be sufficient. Moreover, another kind of practice may be flourishing, probably done by social workers, that is going to look a lot like traditional occupational therapy. In fact, I am on the University of Southern Califotnia's Neighborhood Outreach Board, which reviews proposals for community outreach programs. Recently, I reviewed 30 proposals—most of which I would label "community-based occupational therapy" projects—for homeless people, for at-risk youth, and for youth in foster care. The programs involved activities like gardening. Some were transitional living programs. Unfortunately, funding for those programs in California is being channeled into social work. Mary Reilly predicted this possibility 30 to 40 years ago. Our profession must retain its professionalism and autonomy and must not surrender to the pressure of third-party payers. We must remain true to our traditional beliefs and convince payers of their importance in health care.

Another strategy is that we can infiltrate health maintenance organizations and can become advocates for the need for occupational therapy. I really think occupational therapy has a lot to offer managed care environments. Fortunately, Gary has developed a very marketable kind of approach that I think can open doors for our profession.

Alexis Henry   I am an educator and I see the jobs that new graduates are taking.
Audience Participant I am also on the board of directors of a community program—a clubhouse model program in central Massachusetts where, of course, no occupational therapists are employed. One of the dilemmas that I see is that the new graduates of my undergraduate program are offered $40,000 to work in geriatrics and acute rehab as their first job, and these community programs pay $25,000 per year. I think that, at least in the way in which occupational therapists are being reimbursed in other areas of practice, community mental health programs cannot compete and attract enough occupational therapists to sustain and expand the role of occupational therapy in those programs.

Sally Schultz   I am in total agreement, and in my closing remarks I will address what I am doing in terms of working in the public schools with severely emotionally disturbed children. In fact, I am not too opposed to what is happening in the psychiatric hospital setting because I think that we have an opportunity to make a difference where real life occurs, and that place is in the community. I am in no way concerned about whether therapists will be paid in community settings, because I firmly believe that the services we have to offer are so profound and good that society will pay for them because they are truly valuable. We have the potential to make that contribution, and I know it can occur.

Hans Jonsson
Audience Participant

If I look at the three theoretical conceptions and models (occupational science, model of human occupation, and occupational adaptation), I can see the focus on different levels without thinking about the different conceptualizations. You are saying that occupation science is really a basic science. You address and focus on the general questions about human occupation. As I look at the model of human occupation, I see it is focused on occupation and on function and dysfunction along with what types of things to address. I can see how you could divide the model of human occupation into different subsystems, and I can see the development of the model of human occupation instruments that try to deal with how you understand the function and dysfunction of this individual (Dee). When I finally look at your occupational adaptation model, I see that it addresses this case, the development and treatment session, and the relative mastery. You have a very simple instrument to measure relative mastery from the individual's point of view, and I think you focus on that measurement. Would you agree with me about this different kind of focus in your model?

Gary Kielhofner   I agree with part of what you say, Hans. The distinction between occupational science and the model of human occupation (as well as other conceptual practice models) is an accurate distinction. What I do not agree with is that the model of human occupation does not focus on process. I think that was at one time a valid criticism of the model. However, the current version of the model has a strong emphasis on the process of therapy as reflected in the chapter on the principles of therapy in the second edition of *A Model of Human Occupation: Theory and Application* (Kielhofner, 1995). That chapter specifically proposes theoretical arguments about the nature of changes that take place in a therapeutic context, while only a beginning, but the focus is clearly there.

Florence Clark   I agree with you, Hans, and I think that these three perspectives are all fleshing out important perspectives on occupation, and I agree with how you have organized them. I was trying to do that, but it wasn't coming together in a coherent order. I think that what you propose makes sense. I do not think that these approaches should be viewed as competitive or conflicting. I think of them as complementary and, fortunately, all of us are focused on aspects of occupation. We need every bit of this work to counteract the "termites of reductionism" that are ravaging practice. All of these approaches are occupation centered and focused.

Sally Schultz   I would like to say that to be juxtaposed with occupational science and the model of human occupation is a position that anyone would find flattering.

Audience Remarks

Audience Participant   One thing that has been stressed is the importance of the context and the person, of the goodness-of-fit between them, and of the way you approach patients from their perspective. I think the other piece that has to be factored in is the goodness-of-fit between the therapist and the theoretical orientation or the way you approach that fit. Sometimes we forget context and try to say that only one theory is true; only one way is right. If we look at what resonates with us, what we feel comfortable with, and what aspects of an approach we want to use, we can look at the different theories while seeing that they would work well if there were a goodness-of-fit between the therapist and that approach.

Audience Participant   Listening to the presentation, we were joking and trying to figure out if the best way to treat this woman would be with a tile trivet, with copper tooling, or with clay. If we used clay, would we throw the clay to get rid of anger, or create a feeling mug that would be more soothing? The point was that when I went to school in 1975, that was the level of discourse within our profession. What we have seen today is an example of how our knowledge has developed. My question thus becomes as follows: "Given the extent that knowledge has developed, is it time, in your opinion, to establish another tier of practitioner?" Maybe this question is related to entry into a master's level, although not necessarily, but with the complexity of knowledge, practitioners need to upgrade their skills of practice to the level that you are all talking about. Don't we need to think about another level of practitioner? We say we work in work, play, and self-care. We don't teach our students work, play, and self-care. Our students do not have courses on what is play, what is work, or what is leisure. Can we upgrade to another level of practitioner?

Florence Clark I am dreaming of offering clinical doctoral degrees, so I definitely think that this knowledge is very complex. At USC right now, the Chair of the Physical Therapy Department maintains that she cannot train physical therapists adequately at the master's level. Yet she is graduating 80 doctors of physical therapy every year. I think that the timing for the clinical doctorate in occupational therapy is right now. The profession is ready to move toward more advanced educational programs with a clinical emphasis. We need a greater investment in master's and doctoral education that is clinically focused at the same time we promote PhD programs in occupational science.

Closing Remarks

Sally Schultz In response to the query "How is the frame of reference linked to education and practice?" I would say that through the integration of occupation and adaptation, this frame of reference serves as both a focus for scholarly research and a focus for treatment. Janette Schkade and I believe that occupational adaptation helps narrow the gap between practice and academia because it is a theoretical perspective that is practice oriented. Occupational adaptation is presented as a framework that is widely applicable to various populations and treatment environments. For example, I am now engaged in doing research in practice treatment settings in which I am developing population-specific practice models at an elementary school where I work with students who have severe behavior disorders. The outcomes from that research are extremely promising. Both undergraduate and master's students work with me in this grant-supported research. For a large forensic psychiatric hospital, we have developed and implemented a practice model that will result in restructuring the entire psychiatric rehabilitation program. The results have been very positive. Other forms of research on occupational adaptation are being done by other faculty members at the Texas Woman's University.

Sally Schultz   The practice of the future will require that therapists be educated to apply the principles of occupational therapy in multiple arenas. Occupational adaptation has the potential to ease the student's ability to succeed in those new domains of practice. I would like to close with this quotation from Sheldon Kopp (1979) that illustrates my understanding of the link between theory, practice, and education (see Appendix A: Occupational Adaptation).

Gary Kielhofner   In my comments I have made several references to the idea of a conceptual practice model, of which the model of human occupation is only one example. The concept of models comes from my book, *Conceptual Foundations of Occupational Therapy* (Kielhofner, 1997), and I want to make a few closing comments that reflect arguments I will make in the upcoming second edition of that text.

Conceptual practice models are, I believe, the context in which the field's theoretical concepts should mainly be developed and in which the field's treatment approaches are laid out. Recently, a lot of discussion in occupational therapy has concerned the role of basic versus applied science. However, distinctions between basic and applied science reflect an outmoded view of how knowledge should develop. I prefer Maxwell's (1992) viewpoint that the separation of theory development and the solving of practical problems are irrational, and they result in much theory of questionable practical value while many pressing human problems remain unsolved. Maxwell proposes a complete rethinking of the nature and purpose of science and scholarship; he proposes that science should proceed in the interest of solving real problems. In a related vein, a recent Carnegie Foundation publication has called for a "scholarship of application" that achieves a meaningful dialogue between theory and its application.

These arguments reflect a growing recognition that it is no longer advisable to separate the search for knowledge from the search for a solution to problems. The idea of a division of labor in which academic disciplines create theory and then professions apply that theory will only perpetuate an unnecessary and unproductive division of theory and application.

Moreover, observations of how theoretical explanation and practice often fail to connect seem to underscore the importance of models that link theoretical explanation and practical action. Since the theory development in conceptual practice models is in response to practical problems, occupational therapists develop those theories as explanations for application. If we are to make sense of the puzzles of practice in a systematic and long-term way, we need to direct our efforts to developing conceptual practice models.

Florence Clark   I would like to make a plug for our new book, *Occupational Science: The Evolving Discipline,* in which Zemke and Clark (1996) state that we no longer agree with the classification of basic and applied science, and we no longer consider occupational science a basic science. We consider it a human science that is concerned with the systematic study of the form, function, and meaning of human occupation in all contexts, including the therapeutic context. So, like it or not, when you do research on occupation, we are going to think that you are doing occupational science.

Afterword

Patricia Crist and
Charlotte Royeen
Co-editors

The future of occupational therapy as a viable health care profession is catapulted forward by capturing this moment in our history. In the rapidly changing health care system, occupational therapy must establish and validate our special contribution to promoting healthy lifestyles and quality of life for the individuals we serve.

These three approaches to occupation—occupational adaptation, model of human occupation, and occupational science—along with others that will emerge will provide a synthesis of our special therapeutic perspectives on the importance of human occupation for health. We thank the presenters, Drs. Sally Schultz, Gary Kielhofner, and Florence Clark, for their cogent, insightful comparative responses to the case study and for the opportunity to further understand the relationship between scholarship and service delivery in occupational therapy.

Both the vitality and viability of occupational therapy will be evident if each one of us, as practitioners, guards against further duplication and reductionism in our services, and instead *advocates putting occupation back into our practice and education*!

Appendix A:
Occupational Adaptation

Sally Schultz

This appendix is intended to illustrate how the occupational adaptation frame of reference incorporates occupation into the therapy process.

Fundamental Beliefs in Occupational Therapy—Corollaries in Occupational Adaptation Frame of Reference

The following corollaries represent three of the most fundamental beliefs of the occupational therapy profession. The corollaries within occupational adaptation illustrate how this frame of reference can be used to integrate theoretical beliefs and assumptions into an organized whole for practice.

Belief: Humans are occupational beings.

Corollary: *The occupational adaptation frame of reference is a way to "name and frame" (think about and communicate about) the occupational nature of human beings.*

———

Belief: Adaptation (change) that occurs through occupation reflects the fundamental process of occupational development leading to competence in occupational functioning.

Corollary: *The occupational adaptation frame of reference is a way to "name and frame" the internal process inherent in the individual's pursuit of competence in occupational functioning.*

———

Belief: Occupational challenge is the stimulus for adaptation. An occupational challenge that makes unusual adaptation demands can lead to occupational dysfunction.

Corollary: *The occupational adaptation frame of reference is a way to "name and frame" an approach to occupational therapy intervention that is individualistic, holistic, and empowering.*

Sally Schultz

Model of Occupational Adaptation— The Process

The Model of Occupational Adaptation Process provides a *normative explanation of how occupation and adaptation interact* given a particular challenge within a "window of time."

When facing an *occupational challenge,* human beings generate an *adaptive response* that produces a result they evaluate as either positive or negative. The outcome of the personal evaluation may or may not affect the way the person responds to that type of challenge in the future.

The other elements in the process model depict the *impact of the other influences on adaptation* (e.g., the person's role and associated expectations; the physical, social, and cultural factors; the person's mental and physical systems.

Therapists use the Occupational Adaptation Process Model to understand how the individual's *adaptive processes* are functioning, to pinpoint where the processes may have blocks, and to identify needed intervention. Some patients or clients can be taught this process and use it to capitalize on their adaptive capacity.

Occupational Adaptation—Distinguishing Aspects of Treatment

Occupational adaptation focuses on enhancement of a *process,* not a discrete skill.

————

Occupational adaptation engages the patient or client not only in treatment planning but also in treatment evaluation.

————

Occupational adaptation requires that all three person systems must be addressed in every treatment session, regardless of the particular setting.

————

Treatment of *person-system deficits* (sensorimotor, cognitive, psychosocial functioning) must be clearly linked with the primary occupational environment and roles that have meaning for the individual.

————

The overriding goal of therapy is to help the patient or client become more adaptive. To accomplish this, the therapist facilitates the internal occupational adaptation process.

Occupational Adaptation—Guide to Practice

The occupational adaptation frame of reference includes a *Guide to Practice* (see *AJOT*, 1992, p. 837). This guide is unique in that it was designed to guide the therapist's thinking rather than to tell the therapist what to do. It keeps the therapist on track by posing the critical questions to ask within each phase of treatment.

The *Guide to Practice* gives the therapist a method to translate the patient's or client's internal adaptive processes into treatment planning and evaluation.

As a generic tool, the *Guide to Practice* is useful regardless of treatment setting or population.

Hallmarks of Occupational Adaptation Intervention—What It Is and What It Is Not

Occupational Adaptation . . .

. . . is *NOT* a collection of techniques or modalities.

. . . is *NOT* intended to replace all other occupational therapy perspectives.

. . . is *NOT* prescriptive regarding specific intervention techniques.

Occupational Adaptation . . .

. . . *is* an organized way of thinking about a patient's occupational function/dysfunction.

. . . *is* a way of focusing intervention to maximize the impact of available time.

. . . *is* a way to intervene that is holistic and empowering.

. . . *is* one guide to client-centered intervention.

Occupational Adaptation—Practice Model: Treating Students with Behavioral Disorders

Core Assumptions

1. Human beings learn best through experiential activity that is meaningful.

2. As Piaget stated, "Knowledge is more than having a set of fact; it is a process, not a state."

3. Knowledge is acquired through adaptive attempts to explore and master the environment.

Sally Schultz

4. Meaningful occupation is the most powerful tool to foster the acquisition of knowledge.

Premise Underlying Occupational Adaptation Intervention

Occupational adaptation focuses on the student's interaction with the occupational environment and the experience of relative mastery in performing the student role. Most students with behavioral disorders (BD) have little satisfaction in their role as a student. Although many of these students have other impairments (person systems: sensorimotor, cognitive, psychosocial deficits), the occupational adaptation frame of reference proposes it is the student's disengagement from the occupational environment that has the greater impact on school failure and social maladjustment. The progressive disengagement stems from the student's inability or misdirected attempt to make successful adaption (i.e., occupational dysadaptation).

An occupational adaptation approach focuses on helping the student generate adaptive responses in which the student perceives the experience of greater relative mastery (efficiency, effectiveness, satisfaction with self and society). The student learns to make new adaptations through occupational activities (school-related, meaningful doing) in which the demand for adaptation is therapeutically directed. Through this process, the potential for generalization, as well as for expanded adaptation, is increased. Occupational adaptation may also provide interventions to improve the person-system deficits (through occupational readiness). However, the target for intervention is to improve the student's adaptiveness through meaningful activity relevant to the student role. Changes in behavior or social skills are not the target of intervention but will occur as a natural by-product of the student's becoming more adaptive and experiencing greater relative mastery.

Effects of Occupational Dysadaptation on Student Role Performance

1. Limited knowledge of impact on occupational environment

2. Limited knowledge of the most basic performance skills

3. Hesitation to begin new tasks

4. Reluctance to ask for help

5. Perpetuation of others' expectation to fail or act out

The rationale that supports occupational adaptation intervention with BD students is the assumption that through therapeutically directed occupations, the student will (a) improve in basic academic skills, and (b) build a foundation on which to create the internal adaptation (changes) necessary to succeed and experience greater relative mastery in the student role.

Significance of Occupational Adaptation with BD Students

Regardless of the number of social skills classes, and reward systems that are implemented, these students will not improve performance until they have additional modes of response and additional patterns of behavior to draw from. Even if person-system deficits are dramatically improved, most students will remain at risk for poor student role performance unless their occupational adaptation process improves as well. Likewise, although the student's performance skills may be improved, if the student remains arrested in the development of adaptive responses, difficulty may persist in occupational performance and the resulting relative mastery.

The acquisition of skills is not enough.

The primary response that BD students have when they experience a challenge to their competencies is avoidance. They typically display one of three behaviors: (a) get angry, (b) quit or shut down, or (c) make a joke of the situation.

Each option is immediately occupationally dysfunctional and potentially occupationally dysadaptive.

The use of meaningful activity that is carefully directed will help the student acquire new options that will increase his or her range of adaptive responses to challenge.

Intervention Methods

Intervention is directed toward effecting *positive change in the student's internal adaptation process* rather than toward outward behaviors.

Therapeutic/Rehabilitative Techniques

1. Put the students in charge of the outcome of their work.
2. Have the students make decisions about their approach to work. Avoid the pitfall of showing them how to do it "right"; let them experience consequences.
3. Have the leader teach basic skills.
4. Have the leader promote the student's developing adaptive, yet effective, ways to experience relative mastery with skills.
5. Incorporate the student's academic skills that are relevant to the activity.

Sally Schultz

Media or Activities

Activities should consist of those that are occupational to the student's age group. The group format should be media with variation in inherent structure and properties. The medium should lend itself to a wide variety of uses, creativity, and problem solving.

Role of Therapist

The therapist's roles should be the following:

- Function as a facilitator.
- Represent the occupational environment.
- Help set parameters and limits congruent with the occupational environment rather than control the students.
- Mediate the degree of the occupational challenge and the demand for adaptation that the student faces.
- Progressively present opportunities for the students to acquire new adaptive responses through self-generation.
- Provide contexts in which students can experience positive roles that are unfamiliar, e.g., going to the office for a ruler, presenting work to lower-grade-level students, demonstrating competencies to other students in the group.
- Teach occupational readiness skills as needed, e.g., how to use a ruler, a computer, a card catalog in the library, words to resolve personal conflicts, consequences of behavior, expectations of the occupational environment.
- Encourage students to be as much in control of the environment as they can negotiate successfully.

Phases of Intervention

Phase I—This phase includes therapist-directed group activities that use a variety of media and that students will find interesting. The therapist will conduct an in vivo evaluation that incorporates skills of manipulating materials and problem solving with materials. A closed group is best; however, one or two students can be added periodically if necessary, with a maximum of six students with one leader. The environment should allow the student to feel supported and encouraged.

Phase II—In this phase students begin to direct the selection of the activities. They begin to assume greater leadership; they start to ask to do things and to learn how to do things in which they are interested. The group leader will incorporate educational relevance into activities to parallel the students' interests.

Phase III—In Phase III the therapist directs the students progressively into more and more academic-oriented work without losing the quality of meaningful activity. Doing art projects may be therapeutic, but focus must remain on student role performance. However, a link can be clearly made between art projects, math skills, problem solving, geography, etc. If the media approach is too far removed from the activities and performance demands of the identified occupational environment and role, the effect on the student's role performance may be compromised. The ideal therapeutic situation is a blend of Phase I and Phase II.

Functional Outcomes

Improved Occupational Role Performance

The following should be measured by the therapist:

- Increased productivity—use of time
- Increased effectiveness—improved quality of work
- Increased satisfaction to self and society—decrease in self-deprecating comments toward self and others; verbalization of belief in ability to perform competently

Changes in Occupational Adaptation Process

The following should be measured by the student:

- Evaluation of the student's own perception of efficiency, effectiveness, and satisfaction to self and others

The following should be measured by the therapist's observation:

- Increased skill in problem solving
- Generalization of skills learned from one context to another
- Generation of novel but effective approaches to problems faced in work
- Greater range of adaptive responses
- Interest in teaching peers how to do the activity
- An increased sense of satisfaction derived from being engaged in productive work

Early Signs of Positive Effects of Occupational Adaptation Intervention

(from research with elementary age students)

1. Students start to get to work immediately after entering room.
2. Students start to monitor each other's behavior: tell other students to not waste supplies; begin to repeat social courtesies taught by the therapist.

Sally Schultz

3. Students assume increased responsibility: ask to help clean up supplies and take them into the office for therapist.

4. Students show increased ability to maintain focus on activity and expect the same from peers.

The goal of occupational adaptation intervention is to positively change the student's internal adaptation process to improve satisfaction with role performance. Meaningful occupation is the tool used to achieve that goal.

Application of the Model of Occupational Adaptation Process—Transition from Student to Clinician

The model of occupational adaptation can be applied to a normative life transition. This application depicts the professional transition from student to clinician. The person is now the student who brings his or her abilities and internal expectations to the occupational challenge of assessing and treating clients and interacting with staff and team members. In this case the occupational environment is represented by the supervisor and others who are setting the external occupational role expectations for the student.

When the student is presented with a particular aspect of the challenge, he or she must generate a response by selecting a personal level of adaptation energy, a pattern of responding, and a class of adaptive behavior to be employed. The student engages personal sensorimotor, cognitive, and psychosocial systems to carry out the response that is seen in the student action. Evaluation of the student's action will be followed by learning and integration of the information in this occupational event into the person systems for future use. The supervisor and others will assess the student's response and determine if the role expectations should be kept the same, relaxed in some way, or increased. Both student and supervisor stand to be affected by their participation in this occupational event.

Occupational Adaptation in Home Health— Guide to Intervention

This guide to intervention is designed for occupational therapy as provided in the home setting. Four phases of intervention are presented: data gathering, intervention plan development, intervention plan implementation, and discharge from occupational therapy. In each phase actions engage both the therapist and the client or family. Likewise, each phase has expected outcomes as a result of the intervention actions. Following this guide, the therapist can develop an intervention plan that involves the client or family throughout the therapy process. The client or family is active and integral to the therapy process and to the gains in occupational functioning.

Reading List

Occupational Adaptation Frame of Reference (theoretical publications)

MacRae, A., Falk-Kessler, J., Juline, D., Padilla, R., Schultz, S., & Schkade, J. K. (in press). Occupational therapy models. In A. MacRae & E. Cara (Eds.), *The clinical practice of psychosocial occupational therapy*. Albany, NY: Del Mar Press.

Pasek, P. B., & Schkade, J. K. (1996). Effects of a skiing experience on adolescents with limb deficiencies: An occupational adaptation perspective. *American Journal of Occupational Therapy, 50,* 24–31.

Schkade J., & Schultz, S. (1992). Occupational adaptation: Toward a holistic approach for contemporary practice, part 1. *American Journal of Occupational Therapy, 46,* 829–837.

Schkade, J., & Schultz, S. (1993). Occupational adaptation: An integrative frame of reference. In H. Hopkins & H. Smith (Eds.), *Willard and Spackman's occupational therapy* (8th ed.). Philadelphia: J. B. Lippincott.

Schkade, J. K., & Schultz, S. (in press). Occupational Adaptation. In M. Neistadt & E. Crepeau (Eds.), *Willard and Spackman's occupational therapy* (9th ed.). Philadelphia: J. B. Lippincott.

Schultz, S. (1992). School-based occupational therapy for students with behavior disorders. In S. Merrill (Ed.), *Occupational therapy and psychosocial dysfunction.* New York: Haworth Press.

Schultz, S., & Bullock, L. (1991). Occupational therapy: A little known, underutilized related service for students with behavioral disorders. In S. Braaten & E. Wild (Eds.), *Programming for adolescents with behavioral disorders.* Reston, VA: Council for Children with Behavioral Disorders of the Council for Exceptional Children.

Schultz, S., & Schkade, J. (in press). Adaptation: Modifying the person/performance transaction. In C. Christiansen & C. Baum (Eds.), *Occupational therapy: Achieving performance needs in daily living.* Thorofare, NJ: Slack.

Schultz, S., & Schkade, J. (1992). Occupational adaptation: Toward a holistic approach for contemporary practice, part 2. *American Journal of Occupational Therapy, 46,* 917–925.

Application of Occupational Adaptation (practice-based publications)

Ford, K. (1995). Occupational adaptation in home health: A therapist's viewpoint. *Home & Community Special Interest Newsletter, 2*(1), 2–4.

Garrett, S., & Schkade, J. K. (1995). The occupational adaptation model of professional development as applied to level II fieldwork in occupational therapy: An exploratory study. *American Journal of Occupational Therapy, 49,* 119–126.

Gibson, J., & Schkade, J. K. (in press). Effects of occupational adaptation treatment with CVA. *American Journal of Occupational Therapy.*

Johnson, J., & Schkade, J. K. *Occupational adaptation: Effect of intervention on mobility problems following a cerebral vascular accident.* Manuscript submitted for publication.

Lipoma, J. B. (1996). Outcome measures: Are we addressing value from the client's perspective? *Home and Community Health Special Interest Section Newsletter, 3*(2), 1–4.

Ross, M. (1994, August 11). Applying theory to practice. *OT Week,* 16–17.

Schultz, S., & Schkade, J. (1994). Home health care: A window of opportunity to synthesize practice. *Home & Community Health Special Interest Section Newsletter, 1*(3), 1–4.

On Challenge (relevant to meaning)

Csikszentmihalyi, M. (1990). *Flow.* New York: HarperCollins.

On Transition (relevant to normalcy of adaptation)

Dr. Seuss. (1990). *Oh, the places you'll go.* New York: Random House.

On a Balanced Lifestyle (implications for adaptation energy)

McGee-Cooper, A. (1992). *You don't have to go home from work exhausted!* New York: Bantam Books.

Appendix B: Model of Human Occupation

Gary Kielhofner

The Assessment of Communication and Interaction Skills

The Assessment of Communication and Interaction Skills (ACIS) is a formal observational tool designed to measure an individual's performance in the area of personal and group communication. To administer the ACIS, the occupational therapist observes the client in a group activity (observation periods are approximately 30 to 60 minutes); it may be possible to observe more than one person during a group. Skills are scored on a 4-point scale (4 = competent, 3 = questionable, 2 = ineffective, 1 = deficit) following the scoring criteria for each item provided in a manual. Comments that describe behaviors for a given rating may be entered on the form.

Simon (1989) developed the first version of the ACIS and studied its interrater reliability. Salamy (1993) made revisions to the ACIS. Salamy then further tested the instrument in a clinical setting. Using Rasch analysis Salamy's study supports the conclusion that the items form a single unidimensional scale (construct validity). Forsyth (1996) provided substantial evidence of the scale validity and utility. Further development of this instrument is anticipated.

References

Forsyth, K. (1996). *Validity of the Assessment for Communication and Interaction Skills*. Unpublished master's thesis, University of Illinois at Chicago.

Forsyth, K., Salamy, M., Simon, S., & Kielhofner, G. (1995). *A user's guide to the Assessment of Communication and Interaction Skills*. Manual published by the Model of Human Occupational Clearinghouse, Department of Occupational Therapy, University of Illinois at Chicago.

Salamy, M. (1993). *Construct validity of the Assessment for Communication and Interaction Skills*. Unpublished master's thesis, University of Illinois at Chicago.

Salamy, M., Simon, S., & Kielhofner, G. (1993). *The Assessment of Communication and Interaction Skills* (Research version). Department of Occupational Therapy, University of Illinois at Chicago.

Simon, S. (1989). *The development of an Assessment for Communication and Interaction Skills*. Unpublished master's thesis, University of Illinois at Chicago.

The Assessment of Motor and Process Skills

The Assessment of Motor and Process Skills (AMPS) (Fisher, 1994) is used to evaluate the quality or effectiveness of the actions of performance (motor and process skills) as they unfold over time when a person performs daily life tasks. The AMPS is a structured, observational evaluation. The AMPS is intended to be administered and

Gary Kielhofner

scored within a 30- to 60-minute period. In most cases, the client completes two or three tasks that take 10 to 20 minutes each to perform. For each task performed, the client is rated on 16 motor skill items and 20 process skill items. These motor and process skill items were derived from theoretical constructs described in the literature and have been validated through research. Numerous studies supporting the validity and reliability of the AMPS are listed below. The results of these validity and reliability studies support the internal consistency of the AMPS motor and process skills scales, the stability of the AMPS measures over time, and the ability of the measures to remain stable when the AMPS is scored by different raters.

References

Fisher, A. G. (1994). *Assessment of Motor and Process Skills* (version 8.0). Unpublished test manual, Department of Occupational Therapy, Colorado State University, Fort Collins, CO.

Fisher, A. G. (1993). The assessment of IADL motor skills: An application of many-faceted Rasch analysis. *American Journal of Occupational Therapy, 47,* 319–338.

The Occupational Performance History Interview

The Occupational Performance History Interview (OPHI) is a semi-structured interview designed to gather an individual's history of work, play, and self-care performance. The instrument can be used with both psychiatric or physically disabled adolescents and adults. The interview consists of 39 recommended questions covering five content areas. The content areas include (a) organization of daily living routines; (b) life roles; (c) interests, values, and goals; (d) perceptions of ability and responsibility; (e) environmental influences.

The interview takes approximately 45 to 60 minutes to complete. The interview is structured to assist the patient in relating his or her life story, with the occupational therapist and patient identifying a "turning point" that divides the interview, and the subsequent life history, into past and present.

The rating form requires the interviewer to quantify the information that was collected during the interview. The interviewer scores 10 items (2 for each of the 5 content areas). Each item is rated on a 5-point scale, indicat0ing the degree of adaptive occupational function the client reports. Finally, a Life History Narrative form is used to report qualitative data from the interview, and a 5-item nominal scale called the Life History Pattern is used to characterize the individual's overall history.

The first study of the OPHI with psychiatric clients found modest test-retest and interrater reliability (Kielhofner & Henry, 1988). Consequently, a second study (Kielhofner, Henry, Walens, & Rogers, 1991) examined interrater stability of the interview. A more recent study (Mallinson, Kielhofner, & Mattingly, in press), rephrased the issues by more closely examining the actual content of the interview and the data it provides. This study yielded implications for the way historical interviews are conducted, including the importance of using narrative-evoking strategies and attention to how patients interpret their lives.

References

Gutkowski, L. (1992). *A generalized study of the revised Occupational Performance History Interview.* Unpublished master's thesis, University of Illinois at Chicago.

Kielhofner, G., & Henry, A. D. (1988). Development and investigation of the Occupational Performance History Interview. *American Journal of Occupational Therapy, 42,* 489–498.

Kielhofner, G., Henry, A., & Walens, D. (1989). *A user's guide to the Occupational Performance History Interview.* Bethesda, MD: American Occupational Therapy Association.

Kielhofner, G., Henry, A., Walens, D., & Rogers, E. S. (1991). A generalizability study of the Occupational Performance History Interview. *Occupational Therapy Journal of Research, 11,* 292–306.

Mallinson, T., Kielhofner, G., & Mattingly, C. (in press). A narrative analysis of the Occupational Performance History Interview. *American Journal of Occupational Therapy.*

The Occupational Questionnaire

The Occupational Questionnaire (OQ) is a pen-and-paper, self-report instrument that asks the individual to provide a description of typical use of time and uses Likert-type ratings of competence, importance, and enjoyment during activities. The OQ asks clients to complete the instrument in two parts. First, he or she completes a list of the activities he or she performs each half hour on a typical weekday. After listing the activities, the client is asked to answer four questions for each activity. The questions ask the client to rate whether he or she considers the activity to be work, daily living tasks, recreation, or rest, and to consider how well he or she does the activities, how important they are to him or her, and how much he or she enjoys doing them. The occupational therapist can use the scores to calculate the quality of waking activities in terms of value, interest, and personal causation, along with the actual

Gary Kielhofner

number of half hours spent in activity. This instrument was pilot tested in a study that was by Riopel (1982) and that was interested in establishing the impact patterns of daily activity had on volition and life satisfaction. This preliminary evidence suggested the OQ had adequate test-retest reliability and concurrent validity. Since that time, little psychometric work has been added, although the instrument has been used extensively in clinical research studies, often to compare the difference in patterns of time use between occupationally dysfunctional clients and their well peers.

References

Smith, N. R., Kielhofner, G., & Watts, J. (1986). The relationship between volition, activity pattern, and life satisfaction in the elderly. *American Journal of Occupational Therapy, 40,* 278–283.

The Role Checklist

The Role Checklist is a self-report checklist that can be used to obtain information about the types of roles that people engage in and that they use to organize their daily lives. This checklist provides data on an individual's perception of his or her roles over the course of a lifetime and also the degree of value, i.e., the significance and importance, that individuals place on those roles. The Role Checklist can be used with adolescent, adult, or geriatric populations.

The Role Checklist asks the client to consider each of 10 roles described on the form. These roles are student, worker, volunteer, caregiver, home maintainer, friend, family member, religious participant, hobbyist or amateur, and participant in organizations. The checklist itself is in two parts. Part One asks the clients to check those roles they have performed in the past, are currently involved in, or plan to perform in the future. In Part Two of the checklist, the clients are asked to indicate how much worth or importance, i.e., how much value, each of the 10 roles has for them. Each role is rated as to whether the person finds it "not at all valuable," "somewhat valuable," or "very valuable." The Role Checklist takes approximately 15 minutes for a client to complete. The occupational therapist is encouraged to remain with the client to answer or clarify questions.

The majority of the psychometric work on the Role Checklist was carried out during the development of the instrument (for details see Oakley, Kielhofner, Barris, & Reichler, 1986). Content validity was established by an extensive review of the literature and a review by a panel of occupational therapists, which resulted in revisions to some aspects of the checklist. Initial measures of test-retest reliability indicated that the instrument was reasonably stable over time with adults.

References

Barris, R., Oakley, F., & Kielhofner, G. (1988). The Role Checklist. In B. Hemphill (Ed.), *Mental Health Assessment in Occupational Therapy.* Thorofare, NJ: Slack.

Barrows, C. (1988). *Stability of self-report measures of volition in bipolar affective disorder.* Unpublished master's thesis, Boston University, Boston, MA.

Oakley, F., Kielhofner, G., Barris, R., & Reichler, R. K. (1986). The Role Checklist: Development and empirical assessment of reliability. *Occupational Therapy Journal of Research, 6,* 157–170.

Pezzulli, T. (1988). *Test-retest reliability of the role checklist with depressed adolescents in short-term psychiatric hospitals.* Unpublished master's thesis, Virginia Commonwealth University, Richmond, VA.

The Self-Assessment of Occupational Functioning

The Self-Assessment of Occupational Functioning (SAOF) and its corresponding children's version were developed out of a belief that collaborative treatment planning between patient and occupational therapist is a prerequisite to effective occupational therapy intervention. The SAOF is a checklist that consists of a series of statements; these statements correspond with the components of the Model of Human Occupation. The patient rates each statement as a strength, as adequate, or as an area needing improvement. Priorities are then identified from among the latter and are listed. The form is designed so that the entire process of self-assessment and setting priorities among goals is represented visually; this organization affords both patient and occupational therapist a quick overview of the patient's level of function. The instrument then becomes the vehicle for a discussion of treatment planning. A collaborative treatment plan is then written in the patient's words.

Two content validity studies have been completed on the adult or adolescent version of the SAOF. These studies indicate that the SAOF is theoretically sound. Occupational therapists can be reasonably sure that the statements represent the concepts of the Model of Human Occupation. A survey was also completed to examine the usability of this instrument in clinical practice. As a result, the instrument was revised to improve its "user friendliness."

References

Baron, K. (1991). *The Self-Assessment of Occupational Functioning: An efficacy study.* Unpublished master's thesis, University of Illinois at Chicago.

Baron, K. B., & Curtin, C. (1990). *A manual for use with the Self-Assessment of Occupational Functioning*. Department of Occupational Therapy, University of Illinois at Chicago.

Reading List on the Model of Human Occupation[1]

Published Works on Psychiatry

Affleck, A., Bianchi, E., Cleckley, M., Donaldson, K., McCormack, G., & Polon, J. (1984). Stress management as a component of occupational therapy in acute care settings. *Occupational Therapy in Health Care, 1*(3), 17–41. (C)

Baron, K. (1991). *The Self-Assessment of Occupational Functioning: An efficacy study*. Unpublished master's thesis, University of Illinois at Chicago.

Baron, K. B., & Curtin, C. (1990). *A manual for use with the Self-Assessment of Occupational Functioning*. Department of Occupational Therapy, University of Illinois at Chicago.

Barris, R. (1986). Occupational dysfunction and eating disorders: Theory and approach to treatment. *Occupational Therapy in Mental Health, 6*(1), 27–45. (C,T)

Barris, R., Dickie, V., & Baron, K. (1988). A comparison of psychiatric patients and normal subjects based on the model of human occupation. *Occupational Therapy Journal of Research, 8,* 3–37. (R)

Bavaro, S. M. (1991). Occupational therapy and obsessive-compulsive disorder. *American Journal of Occupational Therapy, 45,* 456–458.

Borell, L., Gustavsson, A., Sandman, P., & Kielhofner, G. (1994). Occupational programming in a day hospital for patients with dementia. *Occupational Therapy Journal of Research, 14,* 4. (C, R)

Borell, L., Sandman, P., & Kielhofner, G. (1991). Clinical decision making in Alzheimer's disease. *Occupational Therapy in Mental Health, 11*(4), 111–124.

Brollier, C., Watts, J. H., Bauer, D., & Schmidt, W. (1989a). A content validity study of the Assessment of *Occupational Functioning. Occupational Therapy in Mental Health, 8*(4), 29–47. (I,R)

Brollier, C., Watts, J. H., Bauer, D., & Schmidt, W. (1989b). A concurrent validity study of two occupational therapy evaluation instruments: The AOF and OCAIRS. *Occupational Therapy in Mental Health, 8*(4), 49–59. (R)

---

[1]Each citation is coded at the end: C = Clinical Application; T = Theoretical Discussion; R = Research; I = Instrument Development; E = Educational Application.

Brown, T., & Carmichael, K. (1992). Assertiveness training for clients with psychiatric illness: A pilot study. *British Journal of Occupational Therapy, 55*(4), 137–140. (C)

Burrows, E. (1989). Clinical practice: An approach to the assessment of clinical competencies. *British Journal of Occupational Therapy, 52*, 222–226. (C,E)

Clark, F. (1993). Occupation embedded in a real life: Interweaving occupational science and occupational therapy. *American Journal of Occupational Therapy, 47*, 1067–1078.

Cull, G. (1989). Anorexia nervosa: A review of theory approaches to treatment. *Journal of New Zealand Association of Occupational Therapists, 40*(2), 3–6. (C)

de las Heras, C. G., Dion, G. L., & Walsh, D. (1993). Application of rehabilitation models in a state psychiatric hospital. *Occupational Therapy in Mental Health, 12*(3), 1–32.

DeForest, D., Watts, J. H., & Madigan, M. J. (1991). Resonation in the model of human occupation: A pilot study. *Occupational Therapy in Mental Health, 11*(2/3), 57–75. (R)

Doble, S. (1988). Intrinsic motivation and clinical practice: The key to understanding the unmotivated client. *Canadian Journal of Occupational Therapy, 55*, 75–81 (C,T)

Evans, J., & Salim, A. A. (1992). A cross-cultural test of the validity of occupational therapy assessments with patients with schizophrenia. *American Journal of Occupational Therapy, 46*, 685–695.

Fisher, A. G. (1994). *Assessment of Motor and Process Skills* (version 8.0). Unpublished test manual, Department of Occupational Therapy, Colorado State University, Fort Collins, CO.

Fisher, A. G. (1993). The assessment of IADL motor skills: An application of many-faceted Rasch analysis. *American Journal of Occupational Therapy, 47*, 319–338.

Forsyth, K., Salamy, M., Simon S., & Kielhofner, G. (1995). *A user's guide to the Assessment of Communication and Interaction Skills.* Manual published by the Model of Human Occupation Clearinghouse, Department of Occupational Therapy, University of Illinois at Chicago.

Froehlich, J. (1992). Occupational therapy interventions with survivors of sexual abuse. *Occupational Therapy in Health Care, 8*(2/3), 1–25. (C)

Grogan, G. (1991a). Anger management: A perspective for occupational therapy (Part 1). *Occupational Therapy in Mental Health, 11*(2/3), 135–148. (C)

Grogan, G. (1991b). Anger management: A perspective for occupational therapy (Part 2). *Occupational Therapy in Mental Health, 11*(2/3), 149–171. (C)

Gusich, R. (1984). Occupational therapy for chronic pain: A clinical application of the model of human occupation. *Occupational Therapy in Mental Health, 4*(3), 59–73. (C)

Gusich, R. L., & Silverman, A. L. (1991). Basava day clinic: The model of human occupation as applied to psychiatric day hospitalization. *Occupational Therapy in Mental Health, 11*(2/3), 113–134. (C)

Helfrich, C., & Kielhofner, G. (1994). Volitional narratives and the meaning of occupational therapy. *American Journal of Occupational Therapy, 48,* 319–326. (C)

Helfrich, C., Kielhofner, G., & Mattingly, C. (1994). Volition as narrative: An understanding of motivation in chronic illness. *American Journal of Occupational Therapy, 42,* 311–317. (C)

Henry, A. D. & Coster, W. J. (1996). Predictors of functional outcome among adolescents and young adults with psychotic disorders. *American Journal of Occupational Therapy, 50,* 171–181. (R,T)

Henry, A. D., Tohen, M., Coster, W. J., & Tickle-Degnen, L. (1994, July). *Predicting psychosocial functioning and symptomatic recovery of adolescents and young adults following a first psychotic episode.* Paper presented at the Joint Annual Conference of the American Occupational Therapy Association and Canadian Association, Boston.

Hocking C. (1989). Anger management. *Journal of the New Zealand Association of Occupational Therapists, 40*(2), 12–17. (H)

Jacobshagen, I. (1990). The effect of interruption of activity on affect. *Occupational Therapy in Mental Health, 10*(2), 35–45. (R)

Johnson, C. C. (1995). *Changes in leisure performance in the individual recovering from chemical dependency.* Unpublished master's thesis, Rush University, Chicago.

Jonsson, H., Kielhofner, G. & Borrell, L. (1997). Anticipating retirement: The formation of narratives concerning an occupational transition. *American Journal of Occupational Therapy, 51,* 49–58.

Kaplan, K. (1984). Short-term assessment: The need and a response. *Occupational Therapy in Mental Health, 4*(3), 29–45. (I,R)

Kaplan, K. (1986). The directive group: Short-term treatment for psychiatric patients with a minimal level of functioning. *American Journal of Occupational Therapy, 40,* 474–481. (C)

Kaplan, K. (1988). *Directive group therapy: Innovative mental health treatment.* Thorofare, NJ: Slack. (C)

Kaplan, K. L., & Eskow, K. G. (1987). Teaching psychosocial theory and practice: The model of human occupation as the medium and the message. *Mental Health Special Interest Section Newsletter, 10,* 1–5. (E)

Katz, N., Giladi, N., & Peretz, C. (1988). Cross-cultural application of occupational therapy assessments: Human occupation with psychiatric
inpatients and controls in Israel. *Occupational Therapy in Mental
Health, 8*(1), 7–30. (R)

Katz, N., Josman, N., & Steinmetz, N. (1988). Relationship between cognitive disability theory and the model of human occupation in the assessment of psychiatric and non-psychiatric adolescents. *Occupational
Therapy in Mental Health, 8*(1), 31–44. (R)

Kavanagh, M. R. (1990). Way station: A model community support program for persons with serious mental illness. *Mental Health Special
Interest Section Newsletter, 13,* 6–8. (C)

Kelly, Linda. (1995). What occupational therapists can learn from
traditional healers. *British Journal of Occupational Therapy, 58,*
111–114.

Khoo, S. W., & Renwick, R. M. (1989). A model of human occupation
perspective on mental health of immigrant women in Canada. *Occupational Therapy in Mental Health, 9*(3), 31–49. (C,T)

Kielhofner, G. (1995). *A model of human occupation* (2nd ed.) Baltimore:
Williams & Wilkins.

Kielhofner, G. (1997). Conceptual foundations of occupational therapy
(2nd ed.) Philadelphia: F. A. Davis.

Kielhofner, G., & Brinson, M. (1989). Development and evaluation of an
aftercare program for young and chronic psychiatrically disabled adults.
Occupational Therapy in Mental Health, 9(2), 1–25. (C,R)

Kielhofner, G., & Mallinson, T. (1995). Gathering narrative data through
interviews: Empirical observations and suggested guidelines. *Scandinavian Journal of Occupational Therapy, 2,* 63–68.

Kielhofner, G., Mallinson, T. & de las Heras, C. G. (1995). Methods of
gathering. In G. Kielhofner (Ed.), *A model of human occupation: Theory and application* (2nd ed.). Baltimore: Williams & Wilkins.

Lancaster, J., & Mitchell, M. (1991). Occupational therapy treatment
goals, objectives, and activities for improving low self-esteem in adolescents with behavioral disorders. *Occupational Therapy in Mental
Health, 11*(2/3), 3–22. (C)

Lederer, J., Kielhofner, G., & Watts, J. (1985). Values, personal causation
and skills of delinquents and non delinquents. *Occupational Therapy
in Mental Health, 5*(2), 59–77. (R)

Mallinson, T., Kielhofner, G., & Mattingly, C. (1996). Like being stuck
on flypaper: Metaphor and meaning in a clinical interview. *American
Journal of Occupational Therapy, 50,* 338–346.

Matusiak, L. (1995). Three toddlers: A descriptive study of who they are and how they act on the world. Unpublished master's thesis, University of Illinois at Chicago.

Maxwell, N. (1992). What kind of inquiry can best help us create a good world? *Science, Technology, & Human Values, 17,* 205–227.

Moore-Corner, R., & Kielhofner, G. (1996). *A user's guide to the Work Environment Impact Scale.* Monograph distributed by Model of Human Occupation Clearinghouse, Department of Occupational Therapy, University of Illinois at Chicago.

Muñoz, J. P. (1988). A program for acute inpatient psychiatry. *Mental Health Special Interest Section Newsletter, 11,* 3–4. (C)

Muñoz, J. P., Lawlor, M., & Kielhofner, G. (1993). Use of the model of human occupation: A survey of therapists in psychiatric practice. *Occupational Therapy Journal of Research, 13*(2), 117–139.

Nelson, D. (1988). Occupation: Form and performance. *American Journal of Occupational Therapy, 42,* 633–641.

Neville, A. (1985). The model of human occupation and depression. *Mental Health Special Interest Section Newsletter, 8,* 1–4. (C,E)

Neville, A., Kriesberg, A., & Kielhofner, G. (1985). Temporal dysfunction in schizophrenia. *Occupational Therapy Mental Health, 5*(1), 1–20. (C)

Neville-Jan, A. (1994). The relationship of volition to adaptive occupational behavior among individuals with varying degrees of depression. *Occupational Therapy in Mental Health, 12*(4), 1–18.

Neville-Jan, A., Bradley, M., Bunn., C., & Gehri, B. (1991). The model of human occupation and individuals with co-dependency problems. *Occupational Therapy in Mental Health, 11*(2/3), 73–97. (C)

Oakley, F. (1987). Clinical application of the model of human occupation in dementia of the Alzheimer's type. *Occupational Therapy in Mental Health, 7*(4), 37–50. (C)

Oakley, F., Kielhofner, G., & Barris, R. (1985). An occupational therapy approach to assessing psychiatric patients' adaptive functioning. *American Journal of Occupational Therapy, 39,* 147–154. (R)

Pan, A. W., & Fisher, A. (1994). The assessment of motor and process skills of persons with psychiatric disorders. *American Journal of Occupational Therapy, 48,* 775–780. (C, I)

Padilla, R., & Bianchi, E. M. (1990). Occupational therapy for chronic pain: Applying the model of human occupation to clinical practice. *Occupational Therapy Practice. 1*(3), 47–52. (C)

Platts, L. (1993). Social role valorisation and the model of human occupation: A comparative analysis for work with people with learning disability in the community. *British Journal of Occupational Therapy, 56*(8), 278–282. (C)

Price-Lackey, P., & Cashman, J. (1996). Jenny's story: Reinventing one-self through occupation and narrative configuration. *American Journal of Occupational Therapy, 50*(4), 306–314.

Rabinow, P. (1984). *The Foucault reader* (pp. 3–29, 170–265, 331–390). New York: Pantheon Books.

Rust, K., Barris, R., & Hooper, F. (1987). Use of the model of human occupation to predict women's exercise behavior. *Occupational Therapy Journal of Research, 7,* 23–35. (R)

Salz, C. (1983). A theoretical approach to the treatment of work difficulties in borderline personalities. *Occupational Therapy in Mental Health, 3*(3), 33–46. (C,T)

Scaffa, M. (1991). Alcoholism: An occupational behavior perspective. *Occupational Therapy in Mental Health, 11*(2/3), 99–111.

Schindler, V. P. (1990). AIDS in a correctional setting. *Occupational Therapy in Health Care, 7*(2/3/4), 171–183. (C)

Sepiol, J. M., & Froehlich, J. (1990). Use of the role checklist with the patient with multiple personality disorder. *American Journal of Occupational Therapy, 44,* 1008–1012. (C)

Shimp, S. L. (1989). A family-style meal group: Short-term treatment for eating disorder patients with a high level of functioning. *Mental Health Special Interest Section Newsletter, 12,* 1–3. (C)

Smith, H. (1987). Mastery and achievement: Guidelines using clinical problem solving with depressed elderly clients. *Physical & Occupational Therapy in Geriatrics, 5,* 35–46. (C)

Turner, V. (1987). *The anthropology of performance* (pp. 1–122). New York: PAJ Publications.

Velozo, C., Kielhofner, G., & Fisher, G. (1990). *A user's guide to the Worker Role Interview* (Research version). Department of Occupational Therapy, University of Illinois at Chicago.

Watts, J. H., Brollier, C., Bauer, D., & Schmidt, W. (1989). The Assessment of Occupational Functioning: The second revision. *Occupational Therapy in Mental Health, 8*(4), 61–87. (I,R)

Watts, J. H., Kielhofner, G., Bauer, D., Gregory, M., & Valentine, D. (1986). The Assessment of Occupational Functioning: A screening tool for use in long-term care. *American Journal of Occupational Therapy, 40,* 231–240. (I,R)

Weeder, T. (1986). Comparison of temporal patterns and meaningfulness of the daily activities of schizophrenic and normal adults. *Occupational Therapy in Mental Health, 6*(4), 27–45. (R)

Appendix C: Occupational Science

Florence Clark

Table 1. Occupational science: description of what it is and how it is to be used.

It is ...

    ... an academic discipline (as is sociology, for example) concerned with the study of the human as an occupational being.

It is not ...

    ... a frame of reference for treatment.

It does not contain ...

    ... established guidelines for treatment or a prepackaged format for treating patients.

But ...

    ... individual practitioners may draw from knowledge generated in occupational science to inform their clinical reasoning about specific cases.

Table 2. Scholarly works that guided our approach to this case.

Bruner, J. (1990). *Acts of meaning*. Cambridge, MA: Harvard University Press.

Clark, F. (1993). Occupation embedded in a real life: Interweaving occupational science and occupational therapy. *American Journal of Occupational Therapy, 47,* 1067–1078.

Kondo, D. (1990). *Crafting selves*. Chicago: University of Chicago Press.

Lave, J. (1988). *Cognition in practice*. Cambridge, MA: Cambridge University Press.

Rabinow, P. (1984): *The Foucault reader* (pp. 3–29, 170–256, 331–390). New York: Pantheon Books.

Searle, J. (1992). *The rediscovery of the mind*. Boston: MIT Press.

Turner, V. (1987). *The anthropology of performance* (pp. 1–122). New York: PAJ Publications.

Table 3. Broad assumptions of occupational science.

- Engagement in meaningful occupation is essential to health
- The recursive relationship between occupation and narrative shapes personal identity.
- Humans are most true to themselves when they are engaged in meaningful and satisfying occupation.

Table 4. Key concepts drawn from the literature that guided the occupational science-based approach to the case.

1. Resistance to disciplinary practices may indicate the need to counteract the medical model.
2. Different selves are constructed through occupation in the contexts of one's life.
3. The patient's system of meaning, a narrative interpretation of oneself as an occupational being, must be the centerpiece of treatment.
4. Meaningful occupation possesses powerful transformative potential.
5. Patients may be viewed as protagonists in a social drama. Social drama is defined by Turner (1987) as a social crisis in which some kind of breach has occurred and redressive action is needed.

Florence Clark   **Table 5.** Key ideas in considering Dee Jackson's case from an occupational science perspective.

1. A patient may experience resistance to the medical model and disciplinary practices.
   a. We are given the institutional narrative, not Dee's narrative. The institution is controlling her narrative. The therapist doesn't seem interested in hearing about Saudi Arabia.
   b. Medical practitioners are controlling the unfolding of Dee's life. The institution is controlling decisions.
   c. Dee is categorized, classified, and has no voice in the case. Disciplinary practices are used in an attempt to normalize Dee.
2. Different selves are constructed through occupation in the context of one's life.
   a. Dee's personhood has been or is distributed across settings in which she engages in the occupations with her multiple identities (wife, mother, soldier, patient).
   b. To understand the many facets of Dee, we need to understand the cultures in which she has existed (army, civilian hospital, military hospital, home).
   c. Dee can begin the process of self-construction. She is not a fixed personality with certain attributes, characteristics, deficits, etc. Dee's self will remold itself in shifting contexts of power and meaning.
   d. We need to understand the connection between Dee's Saudi Arabia experience and the self she is now experiencing, her history in the army, and even her childhood occupations.
3. The patient's system of meaning, Dee's narrative interpretation of herself as an occupational being, must be the centerpiece of treatment. We need to gain a sense of what has happened to Dee in her terms.
   a. The themes for therapeutic intervention identified by the therapist must be scrutinized, questioned, and even possibly rejected (occupational role disruption, history of maladaptive behavior, inability to formulate future issues).
   b. In the interview process, Dee should be encouraged to talk about Saudi Arabia, since we are given

(continued)

Table 5. Key ideas in considering Dee Jackson's case from an occupational science perspective. (*Continued*)

clues that this experience is on her mind and she wants to talk about it.

c. Through the interview process, the therapist should attempt to get a sense of the following:

(1) How has Dee made sense of her life?

(2) What plot is organizing her experience?

(3) What does she wish to gain in her future, if she has any notion?

(4) How are past events affecting her current understanding of her life?

(5) Where is she in her story of herself as an occupational being at this moment?

(6) Why, after so many years, is she questioning army life now?

4. Meaningful occupation possesses powerful transformative potential.

a. To gain a sense of the occupations with therapeutic valence for Dee, we must understand the impact of the contexts in which she has been (Saudi Arabia, medical hospital, army, etc.).

b. We must identify meaningful themes that could interest Dee in occupation. We extract from the case description that Saudi Arabia, children, and service are possible meaningful themes.

c. To gain a sense of the occupational contexts with therapeutic potential, we need to generate hypotheses about Dee's responsiveness to normative practices. We have gained a sense that Dee is not responsive to group interventions and doesn't, at the moment, want to return to work.

d. "Poor work performance" and "poor focus on work" may be situationally specific (Lave, 1988).

5. Dee must be understood as a protagonist in a social drama.

a. Breach: husband's abandonment and betrayal, Saudi Arabia experience, break in her own narrative of who she is and was becoming

b. Crisis: withdrawal, depression

c. Redressive action: hospitalization, treatment, stock-taking, self-scrutinizing

d. Reintegration, reorganization: return to civilian life, decision about future Dee seeks.

Florence Clark

Table 6. Assessment strategy for Dee Jackson using an occupational science perspective.

1. Conduct hermeneutic interview (ongoing, processual).
2. Observe Dee in natural settings and multiple contexts.
3. Come to understand Dee as an occupational being with situationally specific identities and capabilities.
   a. What were Dee's childhood occupations?
   b. What was Dee's experience in high school, post office, army—positive, negative, or mixed? What were her motives for joining the army? What were her intentions?
   c. How does she conceive of motherhood?
   d. How much of her current "poor performance," as labeled by the therapist, is situationally specific?
   e. Is Dee's husband still in her life?
   f. How are the children doing? Is Dee's mother able to care for them?
   g. What is Dee's civilian life going to consist of: employment, home, finances, support systems, relationships?
   h. How can Dee's vision for herself be realized through occupation?

Table 7. Factors to be considered in the intervention process.

1. We are given the institutional narrative on Dee and must examine it in terms of disciplinary practices.
2. Since we have no other information, our only option is to excavate this narrative to detect clues about Dee:
   a. Who is Dee as an occupational being?
   b. What themes might inspire Dee to engage in occupation?
   c. How is she oriented in relation to past, present, and future?
   d. How does she perceive her current situation and its resolution?
   e. What is interfering with her progress, and why doesn't she seem to be responsive to occupational therapy?

Table 8. Steps that would be taken initially in the intervention process in the case of Dee Jackson.

1. The narrative would be placed in Dee's control; she would write the story of herself as an occupational being in the future. Care would be patient centered rather than institution centered.

2. Dee's narrative of herself as an occupational being would be rebuilt, connecting elements of her past self with her emerging self. She would define the problems to be worked on through engagement in occupation. These activities would focus on the present and immediate past.

3. The therapist would assist Dee in resolving the social drama that has become Dee's life: family life, military life, civilian life.

4. "Occupations are not 'put' in our lives; they are out of our lives." (From Brenda Scroggins' interpretation; Scroggins, 1996). Dee is motivated to work on projects directed toward others and children.

5. Consider a way to "safely" return Dee to her family context if this is what she wants.

6. Use extra structural settings and times in the early stages of intervention; use a highly unregimented, individualized treatment style without pressure to conform.

7. Give Dee the time to work through "the frustrations" and "confusions" she experienced in Saudi Arabia. A concern for the future can come later.

8. Assist* Dee is selecting and engaging in occupations that will help her resolve her situation and move forward in her story of herself as an occupational being:

    a. Create parties for her children or others' children.

    b. Prepare dining experiences for others.

    c. Orchestrate celebrations.

    d. Envision herself as a civilian (magazine searches, etc.).

    e. Create an art book on the meaning of her Saudi Arabia experience.

    f. Create gifts for her children.

    g. Work on seemingly mundane activities that address her current concerns (phone calls, bill paying, household tasks, etc.).

    h. Use ritual to resolve breaches in Dee's story.

Most of these ideas were contained in a paper written by Renee McDannel.

Florence Clark

Table 9. Research questions relevant to the case of Dee Jackson.

1. What is the relationship of narrative and engagement in occupation in the therapeutic process?
2. How can narrative be used as a tool to uncover the occupations of therapeutic value to specific patients?
3. Can this genre of intervention be implemented in existing treatment settings?
4. What is the difference in the quality of recovery from illness (e.g., physical, emotional) following occupational therapy using this model as compared with other models?
5. What changes in occupational therapy education need to be made to enable practitioners to use this approach and be successful at advocating its cost-effectiveness to payers?

Bibliography on Occupational Science

Bruner, J. (1990). *Acts of meaning.* Cambridge, MA: Harvard University Press.

Burke, J. P. (1996). Moving occupation into treatment: Clinical interpretation of "legitimizing occupational therapy's knowledge." *American Journal of Occupational Therapy, 50*(8), 635–638.

Clark, F. A. (1993). Occupation embedded in a real life: Interweaving occupational science and occupational therapy. 1993 Eleanor Clarke Slagle Lecture. *American Journal of Occupational Therapy, 47*(12) 1067–1078.

Clark, F. A., Larson Ennevor, E., & Richardson, P. (1996). A grounded theory of techniques for occupational storytelling and occupational story making. In R. Zemke and F. A. Clark (Eds.), *Occupational science: The evolving discipline* (pp. 373–392). Philadelphia: F. A. Davis.

Clark, F. A., Parham, D., Carlson, M. E., Frank, G., Jackson, J., Pierce, D., Wolfe, A. J., & Zemke, R. (1991). Occupational science: Academic innovation in the service of occupational therapy's future. *American Journal of Occupational Therapy, 45*(4), 300–310.

Clark, F., Zemke, R., Frank, G., Parham, D., Neville-Jan, A., Hedricks, C., Carlson, M., Fazio, L., & Abreu, B. (1993). Dangers inherent in the partition of occupational therapy and occupational science. *American Journal of Occupational Therapy, 47*(3), 184–186.

Fraits-Hunt, D., & Zemke, R. (1996). Games mothers play with their full-term and pre-term infants. In R. Zemke & F. A. Clark (Eds.), *Occupational science: The evolving discipline* (pp. 71–80). Philadelphia: F. A. Davis.

Friedson, E. (1994). *Professionalism reborn: Theory, prophesy, and policy* (p. 194). Chicago: University of Chicago Press.

Hoshmand, L. T., & Polkinghorne, D. E. (1992). Redefining the science-practice relationship and professional training. *American Psychologist, 47*(1), 55–66.

Jackson, J. (1993). *Is there a place for role theory in occupational science?* Paper presented at the American Occupational Therapy Association Annual Conference, Seattle, WA.

Kielhofner, G. (1992). Directions for knowledge development. In G. Kielhofner (Ed.), *Conceptual foundations of occupational therapy* (pp. 168–189). Philadelphia: F. A. Davis.

Kondo, D. (1990). *Crafting selves.* Chicago: University of Chicago Press.

Lave, J. (1988). *Cognition in practice.* Cambridge, MA: Cambridge University Press.

McDannel, R. *Dee's case.* Unpublished manuscript.

Mocellin, G. (1992). An overview of occupational therapy in the context of American influence on the profession: Part 2. *British Journal of Occupational Therapy, 55*(2), 55–60.

Mosey, A. C. (1993). The issue is: Partition of occupational science and occupational therapy. *American Journal of Occupational Therapy, 46*(9), 851–853.

Mosey, A. C. (1994). The issue is: Partition of occupational science and occupational therapy: Sorting out some issues. *American Journal of Occupational Therapy, 47*(8), 751–754.

Ottenbacher, K. J. (1992). Nationally speaking: Confusion in occupational therapy research: Sorting out some issues. *American Journal of Occupational Therapy, 46*(10), 871–874.

Parham, L. D., & Fazio, L. (Eds.). (1997). *Play in occupational therapy for children.* St. Louis, MO: Mosby.

Pierce, D. E. (1997). The power of object play with infants and toddlers at risk for developmental delays. In L. D. Parham & L. Fazio (Eds.), *Play in occupational therapy for children.* St. Louis, MO: Mosby.

Polkinghorne, D. E. (1988). *Narrative knowing and the human sciences* (Parts I, II, & III, pp. 1–70). Albany, NY: State University of New York Press.

Polkinghorne, D. E. (1993). A postmodern epistemology of practice. In S. Kvale (Ed.), *Psychology and postmodernism* (pp. 147–165). London: Sage.

Polkinghorne, D. E. (1996). Transformative narratives: From victimic to agentic life plots. *American Journal of Occupational Therapy, 50*(4), 299–305.

Price-Lackey, P., & Cashman, J. (1996). Jenny's story: Reinventing one-self through occupation and narrative configuration. *American Journal of Occupational Therapy, 50*(4), 306–314.

Rabinow, P. (1984). *The Foucault reader* (pp. 3–29, 170–265, 331–390). New York: Pantheon Books.

Scroggins, B. (1996). *Dee's case.* Unpublished manuscript.

Searle, J. (1992). *The rediscovery of the mind.* Boston: MIT Press.

Turner, V. (1987). *The anthropology of performance* (pp. 1–122). New York: PAJ Publications.

Yerxa, E. J. (1991). Seeking a relevant, ethical, and realistic way of knowing for occupational therapy. *American Journal of Occupational Therapy, 45*(3), 200–204.

Yerxa, E. J. (1993). Occupational science: A source of power for participants in occupational therapy. *Journal of Occupational Science (Australia), 1*(1), 3–10.

Yerxa, E. J., Clark, F. A., Frank, G., Jackson, J., Parham, D., Pierce, D., Stein, C., & Zemke, R. (1989). An introduction to occupational science: A foundation for occupational therapy in the 21st century. In A. J. Johnson & E. J. Yerxa (Eds.), *Occupational science: The foundation for practice* (pp. 1–17). Binghamton, NY: Haworth Press.

Zemke, R. (1989). The continua of scientific research designs. *American Journal of Occupational Therapy, 43,* 551–553.

Zemke, R. (1995). Habits. Lesson 5 in AOTA self-study series. In C. Royeen (Ed.), *The practice of the future: Putting occupation back into therapy.* Bethesda, MD: American Occupational Therapy Association.

Zemke, R., & Clark, F. (1996). *Occupational science: The evolving discipline.* Philadelphia, PA: F.A. Davis.

Addendum A: Occupational Science

Florence Clark

In the first edition of *Infusing Occupation Into Practice* I emphasized that occupational science is an academic discipline, not a frame of reference or treatment model. However, I also suggested that individual practitioners may draw from knowledge generated in occupational science to inform their clinical reasoning as they treat patients. Throughout the first edition, I, with the input of my graduate students, illustrated how a circumscribed set of readings relevant to occupational science could be applied in a practical way to guide clinical decisions in a particular case (Dee's case). I pointed out that the theoretical concepts that we highlighted were unique to the readings we cited, and that we relied on this body of knowledge because we were studying it at that time in an occupational science course. I noted that had our class been reading alternate, although related books, our thinking about this case would likely have in some respects differed. This implies that if years later we were given the opportunity to rethink Dee's case, in all probability our product would be significantly modified based on updated research and scholarship in occupational science.

The original workshop at which we presented our conceptualization of Dee's case was held in April 1996; the first edition of this volume was published in 1997. In October 1997, our study group published the findings of the University of Southern California (USC) Well Elderly Study (Clark, Azem, Zemke, et al., 1997), the largest randomized clinical trial ever conducted on the effectiveness of occupational therapy. I believe the results of this research would have influenced and updated my thinking in relation to Dee's case. The study included 361 elderly (60–89 years of age) Los Angeles residents who received nine months of intervention. Results showed that an innovative occupational therapy program based on occupational science—Lifestyle Redesign—improved health and slowed the declines normally associated with aging. Moreover, these positive health outcomes were sustained six months after the elders completed the clinical trial (Clark, Azen, Carlson, et al., in press) and the intervention was shown to be cost-effective (Hay et al., unpublished manuscript). In thinking about Dee's case, I suspect I would have considered how Dee might have benefited from Lifestyle Redesign.

Florence Clark   Although Lifestyle Redesign was developed for elders, I believe it may have therapeutic promise for nearly every clinical population treated by occupational therapists. However, the approach would need to be tailored to the unique needs of each population or individual. In our manual on Lifestyle Redesign approach, my USC colleagues and I outlined a process for making such modifications (Mandel, Jackson, Zemke, Nelson, & Clark, 1999). At its core, Lifestyle Redesign enables patients and consumers to develop and sustain a customized routine of satisfying and health-promoting activity. The approach is based on four key ideas (Mandel, et al., 1999, p. 31).

1. Experience in occupation produces radiating, not linear, change.

2. Occupational self-analysis is possible.

3. When people understand the elements of occupation, they have the toolkit to redesign their lives.

4. Occupation is the impetus that propels people forward.

See the manual for a detailed description of this state-of-the-art intervention, based on occupational science.

Since the first volume of *Infusion* was published, other key occupational science developments have occurred. Other dissertations in occupational science have been published, with more than 20 completed to date (see list of titles at the end of this chapter). The book *Occupational Science: The Evolving Discipline* (Zemke & Clark, 1996), an edited collection of scholarly papers and research reports, was also published, with many chapters that illustrate applications of occupational science to practice. More recently, Wilcock (1998) published a comprehensive theory on the human need for occupation. Wilcock's work underscores how increased knowledge of occupation can contribute to clinical practice and public health. Further, three issues of the *American Journal of Occupational Therapy* (Volumes 52 [5 & 6] and 54 [3]) included many articles reflecting an occupational science perspective, and the *Journal of Occupational Science* endures. In the areas of assessment, Meltzer (2000) has developed a useful clinical tool, the *Self-Discovery Tapestry*, which enables therapists to visually chart the key occupations and major life events of consumers. Finally, at USC, the newly established Center for Occupation and Lifestyle Redesign will promote research on the relationship of occupation to health, provide innovative community programs based on an occupational science perspective, and advance the study of occupation through educational offerings. In this Center, cutting-edge occupational science will be applied to state-of-the-art practice.

References

Clark, F., Azen, S. P., Carlson, M., Mandel, D., LaBree, L., Hay, J., Zemke, R., Jackson, J., & Lipson, L. (in press). Occupational therapy for independent-living older adults: Long-term follow-up. *Journal of Gerontology: Psychological Sciences.*

Clark, F., Azen, S. P., Zemke, R., Jackson, J., Carlson, M., Hay, J., Mandel, D., Josephson, K., Cherry, B., Hessel, C., Palmer, J., & Lipson, L. (1997). Occupational therapy for independent-living older adults: A randomized controlled trial. *Journal of the American Medical Association, 278,* 1321–1326.

Hay, J., Luo, R., Azen, S. P., Carlson, M., Mandel, D., LaBree, L., & Clark, F. (in press). Cost-effectiveness of preventive occupational therapy for independent-living older adults. *Medical Care.*

Mandel, D. R., Jackson, J. M., Zemke, R., Nelson, L., & Clark, F. A. (1999). *Lifestyle redesign: Implementing the Well Elderly Program.* Rockville, MD: American Occupational Therapy Association.

Meltzer, P. (2000). *Self-discovery tapestry* [Instrument]. Redondo Beach, CA: Life Course Publishing.

Zemke, R., & Clark, F. (Eds.). (1996). *Occupational science: The evolving discipline.* Philadelphia: F. A. Davis.

Dissertation Titles

Blanche, E. (1998). Play and process.

Fanchiang, S. P. (1999). Participation in occupations and quality of life in individuals with Parkinson's disease.

Farnworth, L. (1999). The time use and subjective experience of occupations of young male and female legal offenders.

Florey, L. (1998). Summer camp as a transformative experience.

Jackson, J. (1995). Lesbian identities, daily occupations, and health care experiences.

Kao, C. C. (2000). Motivational orientation, achievement, and school-related occupations in Taiwanese gifted children.

Kennedy, B. (1998). Thinking, feeling, and doing: Health and mind-body-environment interactions in daily occupations of women with HIV/AIDS.

Knox, S. (1997). Play and play styles of preschool children.

Krishnagiri, S. (1994). The occupation of mate selection.

Larson, E. (1996). Embracing paradox: The daily experience and subjective well-being of Mexican-origin mothers parenting children with disabilities.

Lo, J. (1994). The relationship between affective experiences during daily occupations and subjective well-being measures.

Ludwig, F. (1995). The use and meaning of routine in women over seventy years of age.

McHugh Pendleton, H. (1998). Establishment and sustainment of friendships of women with physical disability: The role of participation in occupation.

Meltzer, P. (1997). The Self Discovery Tapestry Instrument used by midlife women who are changing occupations through higher education.

Pierce, D. (1996). Conceptualizing infant object play: Development of temporal and spatial negotiation from one to eighteen months.

Primeau, L. (1995). Orchestration of work and play within families.

Russel, E. (1999). Career change in mothers of children with disabilities.

Segal, R. (1995). Family adaptation to a child with attention deficit hyperactivity disorder.

White, J., Jr. (1999). Occupation and Adaptation in Ritual Transformation: An ethnographic study of ten people with disabilities using Title I of the ADA to fight employment discrimination.

Wood, W. (1995). Environmental influences upon the relationship of engagement in occupation to adaptation among captive chimpanzees.

Wright, J. (1995). Occupational restructuring by and selected psychological characteristics of older adults after the death of their spouse.

Updated Bibliography

Azen, S., Palmer, J., Carlson, M., Mandel, D., Cherry, B. J., Fanchiang, S. P., Jackson, J., & Clark, F. (1999). Psychometric properties of a Chinese translation of the SF-36 Health Survey Questionnaire in the well elderly study. *Journal of Aging and Health, 11*(2), 240–251.

Carlson, M., Young, B., & Clark, F. (1998). Practical contributions of occupational science to the art of successful aging: How to sculpt a meaningful life in older adulthood. *Journal of Occupational Science, 5*(3), 107–118.

Carlson, M., Fanchiang, S. P., Zemke, R., & Clark, F. (1996). A meta-analysis of the effectiveness of occupational therapy for the elderly. *American Journal of Occupational Therapy, 50*, 89–98.

Clark, F., Azen, S. P., Carlson, M., Mandel, D., LaBree, L., Hay, J., Zemke, R., Jackson, J., & Lipson, L. (in press). Occupational therapy for independent-living older adults: Long-term follow-up. *Journal of Gerontology: Psychological Sciences.*

Clark, F., Azen, S. P., Zemke, R., Jackson, J., Carlson, M., Hay, J., Mandel, D., Hay, J., Josephson, K., Cherry, B., Hessel, C., Palmer, J. & Lipson, L. (1997). Occupational therapy for independent-living older adults: A randomized controlled trial. *Journal of the American Medical Association, 278*, 1321–1326.

Clark, F., Carlson, M. & Polkinghorne, D. (1997). The issue is: The legitimacy of life history and narrative approaches in the study of occupation. *American Journal of Occupatonal Therapy, 51*, 313–317.

Clark, F., Carlson, M., Zemke, R., Frank, G., Patterson, K., Larson-Ennevor, B., Rankin-Martinez, A., Hobson, L., Crandall, J., Mandel, D., and Lipson, L. (1996). Life domains and adaptive strategies of a group of low-income well older adults. *American Journal of Occupational Therapy, 50*, 99–108.

Hay, J., Luo, R., Azen, S. P., Carlson, M., Mandel, D., LaBree, L., Clark, F. (in press). Cost-effectiveness of preventive occupational therapy for independent-living older adults. *Medical Care*.

Jackson, J., Carlson, M., Mandel, D., Zemke, R., & Clark, F. (1998). Occupation in lifestyle redesign: The Well Elderly Study occupational therapy program. *American Journal of Occupational Therapy, 52*, 326–336.

Jackson, J., Kennedy, B. L., Mandel, D., Carlson, M., Cherry, B., Fanchiang, S. P., Ding, L., Zemke, R., Azen, S., LaBree, L., & Clark, F. (2000). Derivation and pilot assessment of a health promotion program for Mandarin speaking Chinese older adults. *International Journal of Aging and Human Development, 50,* 127–149.

Mandel, D. R., Jackson, J. M., Zemke, R., Nelson, L., & Clark, F. A. (1999). *Lifestyle redesign: Implementing the Well Elderly Program.* Rockville, MD: American Occupational Therapy Association.

Meltzer, P. (2000). *Self-discovery tapestry* [Instrument].Redondo Beach, CA: Life Course Publishing.

Snyder, C., Clark, F., Masunaka-Noriega, M., & Young, B. (1998). Los Angeles street kids: New occupations for life program. *Journal of Occupational Science, 5*(3), 133–139.

Wilcock, A. (1998). *An occupational perspective on health.* Thorofare, NJ: Slack, Inc.

Zemke, R., & Clark, F. (Eds.). (1996). *Occupational science: An evolving discipline.* Philadelphia: F. A. Davis.

Addendum B: Model of Human Occupation

Gary Kielhofner

The Model of Human Occupation (MOHO) has evolved significantly since the first edition of *Infusing Occupation into Practice.* Two of the most important advances have been the further development of the assessment discussed in the case study and the establishment of the MOHO Clearinghouse, set up with the mission to

Gary Kielhofner   enhance occupational therapy practice through the development, testing, and dissemination of knowledge related to the model. The Clearinghouse aims to foster the development of occupational therapy theory by promoting scholarly dialogue among occupational therapists.

The MOHO Clearinghouse

The Clearinghouse, located within the Department of Occupational Therapy, College of Health & Human Development Sciences at the University of Illinois at Chicago, maintains a library of published and unpublished materials related to the Model of Human Occupation. The Clearinghouse is responsible for developing manuals and videotapes that apply the concepts of MOHO to:

- clinical instruments,
- clinical programs, and
- clinical issues.

The Clearinghouse Web site: http://www.uic.edu/hsc/acad/cahp/OT/MOHOC, features the following:

- a listing of MOHO-related workshops and events worldwide
- a comprehensive listing of published articles that examine or otherwise use concepts from the Model of Human Occupation
- current progress on ongoing research projects for collaborators
- a place to sign up as a MOHO research collaborator
- a link to the MOHO listserv so that you can join a discussion group with other occupational therapists on the Model of Human Occupation

MOHO assessments are sold through AOTA. You can order the assessments directly through AOTA's publishing division by using the Web site order form.

We would like to hear from you. Please direct any comments to mohoc@uic.edu

Updated Bibliography

Adelstein, L. A., Barnes, M. A., Murray-Jensen, F., & Skaggs, C. B. (1989). A broadening frontier: Occupational therapy in mental health programs for children and adolescents. *Mental Health Special Interest Section Newsletter, 12,* 2–4.

Arnsten, S. M. (1990). Intrinsic motivation. *American Journal of Occupational Therapy, 44,* 462–463.

Baron, K. (1987). The model of human occupation: A newspaper treatment group for adolescents with a diagnosis of conduct disorder. *Occupational Therapy in Mental Health, 7*(2), 89–104.

Baron, K. (1989). Occupational therapy: A program for child psychiatry. Mental Health Special Interest Section Newsletter, 12, 6–7.

Baron, K. B., & Littleton, M. J. (1999). The model of human occupation: A return to work case study. *Work: A Journal of Prevention, Assessment & Rehabilitation, 12*(1), 37–46.

Barrett, L., Beer, D., & Keilhofner, G. (1999). The importance of volitional narrative in treatment: An ethnographic case study in a work program. *Work: A Journal of Prevention, Assessment & Rehabilitation, 12*(1), 79–92.

Barris, R. (1982). Environmental interactions: An extension of the model of human occupation. *American Journal of Occupational Therapy, 36*, 637–644.

Barris, R. (1986). Activity: The interface between person and environment. *Physical and Occupational Therapy in Geriatrics, 5*(2), 39–49.

Barris, R., Kielhofner, G., Burch, R. M., Gelinas, I., Klement, M., & Schultz, B. (1986). Occupational function and dysfunction in three groups of adolescents. *Occupational Therapy Journal of Research, 6*, 301–317.

Barrow, C. (1996). Clinical interpretation of "Predictors of functional outcome among adolescents and young adults with psychotic disorders." *American Journal of Occupational Therapy, 50*, 182–183.

Behnke, C., & Fetkovich, M. (1984). Examining the reliability and validity of the Play History. *American Journal of Occupational Therapy, 38*, 94–100.

Biernacki, S. D. (1993). Reliability of the Worker Role Interview. *American Journal of Occupational Therapy, 47*, 797–803.

Blakeney, A. (1985). Adolescent development: An application to the model of human occupation. *Occupational Therapy in Health Care, 2*(3), 19–40.

Bledsoe, N. P., & Shepherd, J. T. (1982). A study of reliability and validity of a Preschool Play Scale. *American Journal of Occupational Therapy, 36*, 783–788.

Bränholm, I., & Fugl-Meyer, A. R. (1992). Occupational role preferences and life satisfaction. *Occupational Therapy Journal of Research, 12*, 159–171.

Braveman, B. (1999). The model of human occupation and prediction of return to work: A review of related empirical research. *Work: a Journal of Prevention, Assessment & Rehabilitation 12*(1), 13–23.

Bridgett, B. (1993). Occupational therapy evaluation for patients with eating disorders. *Occupational Therapy in Mental Health, 12*, 79–89.

Bridle, M. J., Lynch, K. B., & Quesenberry, C. M. (1990). Long-term function following the central cord syndrome. *Paraplegia, 28*, 178–185.

Broadley, H. (1991). Assessment guidelines based on the model of human occupation. *World Federation of Occupational Therapists: Bulletin, 23,* 34–35.

Burke, J. P. (1988). Commentary: Combining the model of human occupation with cognitive disability theory. *Occupational Therapy in Mental Health, 8*(2), xi–xiii.

Burke, J. P., Clark, F., Dodd, C., & Kawamoto, T. (1987). Maternal role preparation: A program using sensory integration, infant–mother attachment, and occupational behavior perspectives. *Occupational Therapy in Health Care, 4*(2), 9–21.

Burton, J. E. (1989). The model of human occupation and occupational therapy practice with elderly patients, Part 1: Characteristics of aging. *British Journal of Occupational Therapy, 52,* 215–218.

Burton, J. E. (1989). The model of human occupation and occupational therapy practice with elderly patients, Part 2: Application. *British Journal of Occupational Therapy, 52,* 219–221.

Cermak, S. A., & Murray, E. (1992). Nonverbal learning disabilities in the adult framed in the model of human occupation. In N. Katz. (Ed.), *Cognitive rehabilitation: Models for intervention in occupational therapy* (pp. 258–291). Stoneham, MA: Butterworth-Heinemann.

Chen, C., Neufeld, P. S., Feely, C. A., & Skinner, C. S. (1999). Factors influencing compliance with home exercise programs among patients with upper-extremity impairment. *American Journal of Occupational Therapy, 53*(2), 171–180.

Chern, J., Kielhofner, G., de las Heras, C., & Magalhaes, L. (1996). The volitional questionnaire: Psychometric development and practical use. *American Journal of Occupational Therapy, 50,* 516–525.

Coster, W. J., & Jaffe, L. E. (1991). Current concepts of children's perceptions of control. *American Journal of Occupational Therapy, 45,* 19–25.

Cubie, S., & Kaplan, K. (1982). A case analysis method for the model of human occupation. *American Journal of Occupational Therapy, 36,* 645–656.

Curtin, C. (1990). Research on the model of human occupation. *Mental Health-Special Interest Section Newsletter, 13,* 3–5.

Curtin, C. (1991). Psychosocial intervention with an adolescent with diabetes using the model of human occupation. *Occupational Therapy in Mental Health, 11*(2/3), 23–36.

Davies Hallet, J., Zasler, N., Maurer, P., & Cash, S. (1994). Role change after traumatic brain injury in adults. *American Journal of Occupational Therapy, 48,* 241–246.

DePoy, E. (1990). The TBIIM: An intervention for the treatment of individuals with traumatic brain injury. *Occupational Therapy in Health Care, 7*(1), 55–67.

DePoy, E., & Burke, J. P. (1992). Viewing cognition through the lens of the model of human occupation. In N. Katz, (Ed.), Cognitive rehabilitation: Models for intervention in occupational therapy (pp. 240–257). Stoneham, MA: Butterworth-Heinemann.

Dickerson, A. E., & Oakely, F. (1995). Comparing the roles of community-living persons and patient populations. *American Journal of Occupational Therapy, 49*, 221–228.

Dion, G. L., Lovely, S. & Skerry, M. (1996). A comprehensive psychiatric rehabilitation approach to severe and persistent mental illness in the public sector. In S. M. Soreff (Ed.), *Handbook for the Treatment of the Mentally Ill.*

Doble, S. E. (1991). Test-retest and inter-rater reliability of a process skills assessment. *Occupational Therapy Journal of Research, 11*, 8–23.

Doughton, K. J. (1996). Hidden talents. *OT Week, 10* (26), 19–20.

Duchek, J. M. & Thessing, V. (1996). Is the use of life history and narrative in clinical practice fundable as research? *American Journal of Occupational Therapy, 50*, 393–396.

Duellman, M. K., Barris, R., & Kjelhofner, G. (1986). Organized activity and the adaptive status of nursing home residents. *American Journal of Occupational Therapy, 40*, 618–622.

Dyck, I. (1992). The daily routines of mothers with young children: Using a socio-political model in research. *Occupational Therapy Journal of Research, 12*, 17–34.

Ebb, E. W., Coster, W., & Duncombe, L. (1989). Comparison of normal and psychosocially dysfunctional male adolescents. *Occupational Therapy in Mental Health, 9*(2), 53–74.

Egan, M., Warren, S. A., Hessel, P. A., & Gilewich, G. (1992). Activities of daily living after hip fracture: Pre- and post discharge. *Occupational Therapy Journal of Research, 12*, 342–356.

Elliott, M., & Barris, R. (1987). Occupational role performance and life satisfaction in elderly persons. *Occupational Therapy Journal of Research, 7*, 215–224.

Esdaile, S. A. (1996). A play-focused intervention involving mothers of preschoolers. *American Journal of Occupational Therapy, 50*, 113–123.

Esdaile, S. A., & Madill, H. M. (1993). Causal attributions: Theoretical considerations and their relevance to occupational therapy practice and education. *British Journal of Occupational Therapy, 56*(9), 330–334.

Fidler, G. S. (1996). Life-style performance: From profile to conceptual model. *American Journal of Occupational Therapy, 50*, 139–147.

Fischer, G. S. (1999). Administration and application of the worker role interview: Looking beyond functional capacity. *Work: A Journal of Prevention, Assessment & Rehabilitation, 12*(1), 25–36.

Fitts, H., & Howe, M. (1987). Use of leisure time by cardiac patients. *American Journal of Occupational Therapy, 41,* 583–589.

Forsyth, K., Lai, J., & Kielhofner, G. (1999). The assessment of communication and interaction skills (ACIS): Measurement properties. *British Journal of Occupational Therapy, 62*(2), 69–74.

Fossey, E. (1996). Using the occupational performance history interview (OPHI): Therapists' reflections. *British Journal of Occupational Therapy, 59*(5), 223–228.

Furst, G., Gerber, L., Smith, C., Fisher, S., & Shulman, B. (1987). A program for improving energy conservation behaviors in adults with rheumatoid arthritis. *American Journal of Occupational Therapy, 41,* 102–111.

Gage, M., Noh, S., Polatajko, H., & Kaspar, V. (1994). Measuring perceived self-efficacy in occupational therapy. *American Journal of Occupational Therapy, 48,* 783–790.

Gage, M., & Polatajko, H. (1994). Enhancing occuaptional performance through an understanding of perceived self-efficacy. *American Journal of Occupational Therapy, 48,* 452–461.

Gerardi, S. M. (1996). The management of battle fatigued soldiers: an occupational therapy model. *Military Medicine, 161*(8), 483–488.

Gerber, L., & Furst, G. (1992). Validation of the NIH Activity Record: A quantitative measure of life activities. *Arthritis Care and Research, 5,* 81–86.

Gerber, L., & Furst, G. (1992). Scoring methods and application of the Activity Record (ACTRE) for patients with musculoskeletal disorders. *Arthritis Care and Research, 5,* 151–156.

Gregory, M. (1983). Occupational behavior and life satisfaction among retirees. *American Journal of Occupational Therapy, 37,* 548–553.

Haglund, L., & Henriksson, C. (1994). Testing a Swedish version of OCAIRS on two different patient Groups. *Scandinavian Journal of Caring Sciences, 8,* 223–230.

Haglund, L., & Kjellberg, A. (1999). A critical analysis of the model of human occupation. *Canadian Journal of Occupational Therapy, 66*(2), 102–108.

Hammel, J. (1999). The Life Rope: A transactional approach to exploring worker and life role development. *Work: a Journal of Prevention, Assessment & Rehabilitation, 12*(1), 47–60.

Harrison, H., & Kielhofner, G. (1986). Examining reliability and validity of the Preschool Play Scale with handicapped children. *American Journal of Occupational Therapy, 40,* 167–173.

Henriksson, C. M. (1993). Long-term effects of fibromyalgia on everyday life. *Rheumatology, 23*(1), 36–41.

Henriksson, C., Gundmark, I., Bengsston, A., & Ek, A. C. (1992). Living with fibromyalgia: Consequences for everyday life. *Clinical Journal of Pain, 8,* 138–144.

Henry, A. D., & Coster, W. J. (1997). Competency beliefs and occupational role behavior among adolescents: Explication of the personal causation construct. *American Journal of Occupational Therapy, 51*(4), 267–276.

Heras, C. G., de las Dion, G. L., & Walsh, D. (1993). Application of rehabilitation models in a state psychiatric hospital. *Occupational Therapy in Mental Health, 12*(3), 1–32.

Hocking C. (1989). Anger management. *Journal of the New Zealand Association of Occupational Therapists, 40*(2), 12–17.

Hubbard, S. (1991). Towards a truly holistic approach to occupational therapy. *British Journal of Occupational Therapy, 54*(11), 415–418.

Hurff, J. M. (1984). Visualization: A decision-making tool for assessment and treatment planning. *Occupational Therapy in Health Care, 1*(2), 3–23.

Jackoway, I., Rogers, J., & Snow, T. (1987). The role change assessment: An interview tool for evaluating older adults. *Occupational Therapy in Mental Health, 7*(1), 17–37.

Jongbloed, L. (1994). Adaptation to a stroke: The experience of one couple. *American Journal of Occupational Therapy, 48,* 1006–1013.

Jonsson, H. (1993). The retirement process in an occupational perspective: A review of literature and theories. *Physical and Occupational Therapy in Geriatrics, 3,* 1–20.

Jonsson, H., Kielhofner, G., Borell, L. (1997). Anticipating retirement: The formation of narratives concerning an occupational transition. *American Journal of Occupational Therapy, 51,* 49–56.

Josephsson, S., Backman, L., Borell, L., Hygard, L., et al. (1995). Effectiveness of an intervention to improve occupational performance in dementia. *Occupational Therapy Journal of Research, 15,* 36–49.

Josephsson, S., Bäckman, L., Borell, L., Bernspång, B., Nygård, L., & Rönnberg, L. (1993). Supporting everyday activities in dementia: An intervention study. *International Journal of Geriatric Psychiatry, 8,* 395–400.

Jungersen, K. (1992). Culture, theory, and the practice of occupational therapy in New Zealand/Aotearoa. *American Journal of Occupational Therapy, 46,* 745–750.

Kaplan, K., & Kielhofner, G. (1989). *Occupational Case Analysis Interview and Rating Scale.* Thorofare, NJ: Slack.

Katz, N. (1985). Occupational therapy's domain of concern: Reconsidered. *American Journal of Occupational Therapy, 39,* 518–524.

Katz, N. (1988). Introduction to the Collection (MOHO). *Occupational Therapy in Mental Health, 8*(1), 1–6. (Note: Accompanies Katz, et. al., 1988).

Katz, N. (1988). Interest checklist: A factor analytical study. *Occupational Therapy in Mental Health, 8* (1), 45–56.

Kavanaugh, J. & Fares, J. (1995). Using the model of human occupation with homeless mentally ill patients. *British Journal of Occupational Therapy, 58*(10), 419–422.

Kielhofner, G. (1980). A model of human occupation (Part 2). Ontogenesis from the perspective of temporal adaptation. *American Journal of Occupational Therapy, 34,* 657–663.

Kielhofner, G. (1980). A model of human occupation (Part 3). Benign and vicious cycles. *American Journal of Occupational Therapy, 34,* 731–737.

Kielhofner, G. (1984). An overview of research on the model of human occupation. *Canadian Journal of Occupational Therapy, 51,* 59–67.

Kielhofner, G. (1986). A review of research on the model of human occupation (Part 1). *Canadian Journal of Occupational Therapy, 53,* 69–74.

Kielhofner, G. (1986). A review of research on the model of human occupation (Part 2). *Canadian Journal of Occupational Therapy, 53,* 129–134.

Kielhofner, G. (1992). The future of the profession of occupational therapy: Requirements for developing the field's knowledge base. *Journal of Japanese Association of Occupational Therapists, 11,* 112–129.

Kielhofner, G. (1999). Guest-editorial. *Work: a Journal of Prevention, Assessment & Rehabilitation, 12(1),* 1.

Kielhofner, G., Barris, R., & Watts, J. (1982). Habits and habit dysfunction: A clinical perspective for psychosocial occupational therapy. *Occupational Therapy in Mental Health, 2,* (2), 1–21.

Kielhofner, G., Braveman, B., Baron, K., Fischer, G., Hammel, J., & Littleton, M. (1999). The model of human occupation: Understanding the worker who is injured or disabled. *Work: a Journal of Prevention, Assessment & Rehabilitation 12*(1), 3–11.

Kielhofner, G., & Burke, J. (1980). A model of human occupation (Part 1). Conceptual framework and content. *American Journal of Occupational Therapy, 34,* 572–581.

Kielhofner, G., Burke, J., & Heard Igi, C. (1980). A model of human occupation (Part 4). Assessment and intervention. *American Journal of Occupational Therapy, 34,* 777–788.

Kielhofner, G., & Fisher, A. (1991). Mind-brain-body relationships. In A. G. Fisher, E. A. Murray, & A. C. Bundy, (Eds). *Sensory integration: Theory and practice* . (pp. 27–45). Philadelphia: F. A. Davis.

Kielhofner, G. & Forsyth, K. (1997). The model of human occupation: An overview of current concepts. *British Journal of Occupational Therapy, 60*(3), 103–110.

Kielhofner, G., Harlan, B., Bauer, D., & Maurer, P. (1986). The reliability of a historical interview with physically disabled respondents. *American Journal of Occupational Therapy, 40,* 551–556.

Kielhofner, G., & Henry, A. D. (1988). Development and investigation of the Occupational Performance History Interview. *American Journal of Occupational Therapy, 42,* 489–498.

Kielhofner, G., Henry, A., & Walens, D. (1989). A user's guide to the Occupational Performance History Interview. Rockville, MD: American Occupational Therapy Association.

Kielhofner, G., Henry, A., Walens, D., & Rogers E. S. (1991). A generalizability study of the Occupational Performance History Interview. *Occupational Therapy Journal of Research, 11,* 292–306.

Kielhofner, G., Lai, J. S., Olson, L., Haglund, L., Ekbadh, E., & Hedlund, M. (1999). Psychometric properties of the work environment impact scale: A cross-cultural study. *Work: a Journal of Prevention, Assessment & Rehabilitation, 12*(1), 71–77.

Kielhofner, G., & Nicol, M. (1989). The model of human occupation: A developing conceptual tool for clinicians. *British Journal of Occupational Therapy, 52,* 210–214.

Krefting, L. (1985). The use of conceptual models in clinical practice. *Canadian Journal of Occupational Therapy, 52,* 173–178.

Kyle, T., & Wright, S. (1996). Reflecting the model of human occupation in occupational therapy documentation. *Canadian Journal of Occupational Therapy 63*(3), 192–196.

Larsson, M., & Braholm, I. B. (1996). An approach to goal-planning in occupational therapy and rehabilitation. *Scandinavian Journal of Occupational Therapy, 3,* 14–19.

Levine, R. (1984). The cultural aspects of home care delivery. *American Journal of Occupational Therapy, 38,* 734–738.

Levine, R. E., & Gitlin, L. N. (1990). Home adaptations for persons with chronic disabilities: An educational model. *American Journal of Occupational Therapy, 44,* 923–929.

Levine, R. E., & Gitlin, L. N. (1993). A model to promote activity competence in elders. *American Journal of Occupational Therapy, 47,* 147–153.

Lycett, R. (1992). Evaluating the use of an occupational assessment with elderly rehabilitation patients. *British Journal of Occupational Therapy, 55* (3), 343–346.

Lynch, K., & Bridle, M. (1993). Construct validity of the Occupational Performance Interview. *Occupational Therapy Journal of Research, 13*, 231–240.

Lyons, M. (1984). Shaping up: The model of human occupation as a guide to practice. *Proceedings of the 13th Federal Conference of the Australian Association of Occupational Therapists, 2*, 95–100.

Lyons, M. (1985). Paradise lost! . . . Paradise regained? Putting the promise of occupational therapy into practice. *Australian Journal of Occupational Therapy, 32*, 45–53.

Maynard, M. (1987). An experiential learning approach: Utilizing historical interview and an occupational inventory. *Physical & Occupational Therapy in Geriatrics, 5*(2), 51–69.

Mentrup, C., Niehaus, A., & Kielhofner, G. (1999). Applying the model of human occupation in work-focused rehabilitation: A case illustration. *Work: a Journal of Prevention, Assessment & Rehabilitation, 12*(1), 61–70.

Michael, P. S. (1991). Occupational therapy in a prison? You must be kidding! *Mental Health Special Interest Section Newsletter, 14*, 3–4.

Mocellin, G. (1992). An overview of occupational therapy in the context of the American influence on the profession (Part 1). *British Journal of Occupational Therapy, 55*(1), 7–12.

Mocellin, G. (1992). An overview of occupational therapy in the context of the American influence on the profession (Part 2). *British Journal of Occupational Therapy, 55*(2), 55–60.

Morrison, C. D., Bundy, A. C., & Fisher, A. G. (1991). The contribution of motor skills and playfulness to the play performance of preschoolers. *American Journal of Occupational Therapy, 45*, 687–694.

Muñoz, J. P. (1988). A program for acute inpatient psychiatry. *Mental Health Special Interest Section Newsletter, 11*, 3–4.

Neistadt, M. E. Methods of assessing clients' priorities: A survey of adult physical dysfunction settings. *American Journal of Occupational Therapy, 49*(5), 428–436.

Nygård, L., Bernspång, B., Fisher, A., & Kielhofner, G. (1994). Comparing motor and process ability of persons with suspected dementia in home and clinic settings. *American Journal of Occupational Therapy, 39*, 689–696.

Olin, D. (1985). Assessing and assisting the person with dementia: An occupational behavior perspective. *Physical & Occupational Therapy in Geriatrics, 3*(4), 25–32.

Park, S., Fisher, A., & Velozo, C. (1994). Using the assessment of motor and process skills to compare occupational performance between clinic and home settings. *American Journal of Occupational Therapy, 48,* 697–709.

Pasek, P. B., & Schkade, J. (1996). Effects of skiing experiences on adolescents with limb deficiencies: An occupational adaptation perspective. *American Journal of Occupational Therapy, 50,* 24–31.

Pizzi, M. A. (1984). Occupational therapy in hospice care. *American Journal of Occupational Therapy, 38,* 252–257.

Pizzi, M. A. (1989). Occupational therapy: Creating possibilities for adults with HIV infection, ARC and AIDS. *AIDS Patient Care, 3,* 18–23.

Pizzi, M. A. (1990). The model of human occupation and adults with HIV infection and AIDS. *American Journal of Occupational Therapy, 44,* 257–264.

Pizzi, M. A. (1990). Occupational therapy: Creating possibilities for adults with human immunodeficiency virus infection, AIDS related complex, and acquired immunodeficiency syndrome. *Occupational Therapy in Health Care, 7*(2/3/4), 125–137.

Puderbaugh, J. K. & Fisher, A. G. (1992). Assessment of motor and process skills in normal young children and children with dyspraxia. *Occupational Therapy Journal of Research, 12*(4), 195–216.

Restall, G., & Magill-Evans (1994). Play and preschool children with autism. *American Journal of Occupational Therapy, 48,* 113–120.

Rosenfeld, M. S. (1989). Occupational disruption and adaptation: A study of house fire victims. *American Journal of Occupational Therapy, 43,* 89–96.

Scarth, P. P. (1990). Services for chemically dependent adolescents. *Mental Health Special Interest Section Newsletter, 13,* 7–8.

Schaaf, R. C., & Mulrooney, L. L. (1989). Occupational therapy in early intervention: A family centered approach. *American Journal of Occupational Therapy, 43,* 745–754.

Schindler, V. J. (1988). Psychosocial occupational therapy intervention with AIDS patients. *American Journal of Occupational Therapy, 42,* 507–512.

Series, C. (1992). The long-term needs of people with head injury: A role for the community occupational therapist? *British Journal of Occupational Therapy, 55*(3), 94–98.

Shimp, S. L. (1990). Debunking the myths of aging. *Occupational Therapy in Mental Health, 10* (3), 101–111.

Sholle-Martin, S. (1987). Application of the model of human occupation: Assessment in child and adolescent psychiatry. *Occupational Therapy in Mental Health, 7*(2), 3–22.

Sholle-Martin, S., & Alessi, N.E. (1990). Formulating a role for occupational therapy in child psychiatry: A clinical application. *American Journal of Occupational Therapy, 44,* 871–881.

Smith, R. O. (1992). The science of occupational therapy assessment. *Occupational Therapy Journal of Research, 12,* 3–15.

Smyntek, L., Barris, R., & Kielhofner, G. (1985). The model of human occupation applied to psychosocially functional and dysfunctional adolescents. *Occupational Therapy in Mental Health, 5*(1), 21–40.

Spadone, R. A. (1992). Internal-external control and temporal orientation among Southeast Asians and White Americans. *American Journal of Occupational Therapy, 46,* 713–719.

Spencer, J., Davidson, H., & White, V. (1996). Continuity and change: Past experience as adaptive repertoire in occupational adaptation. *American Journal of Occupational Therapy, 50,* 526–532.

Stofell, V. (1992). The Americans with Disabilities Act of 1990 as applied to an adult with alcohol dependence. *American Journal of Occupational Therapy, 46,* 640–644.

Tatham, M. (1992). Leisure facilitator: The role of the occupational therapist in senior housing. *Journal of Housing for the Elderly, 10*(2), 125–138.

Taylor, L. P., & McGruder, J. E. (1996). The meaning of sea kayaking to persons with spinal cord injury. *American Journal of Occupational Therapy, 50,* 39–46.

Tham, K., & Borell, L. (1996). Motivation for training: A case study of four persons with unilateral neglect. *Occupational Therapy in Health Care, 10*(3), 65–79.

Velozo, C. A. (1993). Work evaluations: Critique of the state of the art of functional assessment of work. *American Journal of Occupational Therapy, 47,* 203–209.

Viik, M. K., Watts, J. H., Madigan, M. J., & Bauer, D. (1990). Preliminary validation of the Assessment of Occupational Functioning with an alcoholic population. *Occupational Therapy in Mental Health, 10*(2), 19–33.

Watts, J. H., & Brollier, C. (1989). Instrument development in occupational therapy. *Occupational Therapy in Mental Health, 8*(4), ix–xi, 1–5.

Watts, J. H., Brollier, C., Bauer, D., & Schmidt, W. (1989). A comparison of two evaluation instruments used with psychiatric patients in occupational therapy. *Occupational Therapy in Mental Health, 8*(4), 7–27.

Watts, J. H., Brollier, C., Bauer, D., & Schmidt, W. (1989). The Assessment of Occupational Functioning: The second revision. *Occupational Therapy in Mental Health, 8* (4), 61–87.

Watts, J. H., Brollier, C., & Schmidt, W. (1989). Why use standardized patient evaluation? Commentary and suggestions. *Occupational Therapy in Mental Health, 8*(4), 89–97.

Weissenberg, R., & Giladi, W. (1989). Home economics day: A program for disturbed adolescents to promote acquisition of habits and skills. *Occupational Therapy in Mental Health, 9*(2), 89–103.

Wieringa, N., & McColl, M. (1987). Implications of the model of human occupation for intervention with native Canadians. *Occupational Therapy in Health Care, 4*(1), 73–91.

Wood, W. (1995). Weaving the warp and weft of occupational therapy: An art and science for all times. *American Journal of Occupational Therapy, 49* (1), 44–52.

Wood, W. (1996). The value of studying occupation: An example with primate play. *American Journal of Occupational Therapy, 50,* 327–337.

Woodrum, S. C. (1993). A treatment approach for attention deficit hyperactivity disorder using the model of human occupation. *Developmental Disabilities Special Interest Section Newsletter, 16*(1), 1–2.

Wu, C., & Lin, K. (1999). Defining occupation: A comparative analysis. *Journal of Occupational Science (Australia), 6*(1), 5–12.

Yelton, D., & Nielson, C. (1991). Understanding Appalachian values: Implications for occupational therapists. *Occupational Therapy in Mental Health, 11*(2/3), 173–195.

Yerxa, E. J. (1992). Some implications of occupational therapy's history for its epistemology, values and relation to medicine. *American Journal of Occupational Therapy, 46,* 79–83.

Zimmerer-Branum, S., & Nelson, D. Occupationally embedded exercise versus rote exercise: A choice between occupational forms by elderly nursing home residents. *American Journal of Occupational Therapy, 49,* 397–402.

Addendum C: Occupational Adaptation

Sally Schultz

I would like to begin by recognizing the wisdom of the Education Special Interest Section (EDSIS) committee in its continued effort to foster the profession's rigorous examination of its theoretical foundations. Current constraints and demands from the health care arena point to the necessity of steadfast commitment to the profession's core beliefs.

Sally Schultz   I would like to first reflect on the 1996 "Putting Occupation into Education and Practice" workshop and the utility of the resulting monograph *"Infusing Occupation into Practice: Comparison of Three Clinical Approaches in Occupational Therapy."* This is my understanding of the comparison of the three theoretical frameworks: Occupational Adaptation, The Model of Human Occupation, and Occupational Science. Being able to compare the frameworks presented in the monograph leads to an opportunity for discovery. Each of the frameworks is most completely understood when situated in relationship to the other two. I suggest that it is only through such triangulation that one can gain a relative sense of each framework. I encourage the reader to:

1. Identify the relative emphases in each framework. Which concepts or methods assume the greatest prominence?

2. Analyze the "target" of the interventions. What does the framework attempt to effect?

3. Clarify the basis for measuring change. How would one recognize therapeutic outcomes based on the framework?

Next, I would like to revisit the 1996 case study presented in this monograph. Given a fresh reading of the material, and the opportunity to amend, I draw the reader's attention to the overwhelming significance that Occupational Adaptation places on the patient's *adaptive response*. My response to the first question (i.e., my understanding of Dee; assessment of function/dysfunction) is entirely focused on the framework's concept of adaptive response. Given the workshop's time constraints, it was necessary to limit my oral reply to the essential. Not until my most recent reading did I appreciate how much I had concentrated my remarks on a single internal process, designated in the Occupational Adaptation framework as the *adaptive response generation subprocess*. I would like to elaborate on and alert the reader to the significance of this subprocess, which Janette Schkade and I (Schkade & Schultz, 1992) proposed as a structure to describe the method by which human beings drive their own adaptive functions. We proposed that human beings activate their adaptive response *mechanism* (a reservoir of various adaptive capacities) and then generate an *adaptation gestalt* (a plan for use of the sensorimotor, cognitive, and psychosocial abilities) to carry out the collective "adaptive response." In my research, and in that of my colleagues with various populations, we have found that the patient's internal process of generating adaptive responses is perhaps the most pivotal factor affecting treatment.

My focus on the patient's adaptive response continues in the reply to second question. Treatment is organized around assessing and facilitating the patient's adaptive capacity. This is accomplished by engaging her in occupation in which the demand to adapt is sufficiently stimulated, yet within her capability. The emphasis on the adaptive response persists as I address the third question. The projected outcome measures are specific to the frame of reference. That is, the therapist wants to see a change in the patient's ability to generate new adaptive responses and to not only generalize that ability, but to extend it to novel situations.

I will close with my own analysis of the three frameworks as presented here. The most distinguishing feature of the Occupational Adaptation approach is the focus on the patient's internal adaptive processes. The relative emphasis on internal adaptiveness appears to be a significant departure from that of both the Model of Human Occupation and Occupational Science. That is, Occupational Adaptation focuses on affecting the patient's internal process of adaptation with the assumption that when that occurs, performance will improve as a result. Conversely, it appears that the other frameworks' focus is on affecting the patient's occupational performance with the assumption that when that occurs, adaptation will occur as a result. Figure 1 in this addendum clarifies the relationship between these two assumptions. I propose that the therapist's choice to target either adaptiveness or occupational performance will markedly change the course of therapy. I would like to say that I encourage comment on these reflections and appreciate the opportunity to add these perspectives.

Updated Bibliography

Buddenberg, L. A., & Schkade, J. K. (1998). A comparison of occupational therapy intervention approaches for older patients after hip fracture. *Topics in Geriatric Rehabilitation, 13*(4), 52–68. *(This clinical study demonstrates the importance of personally chosen activity).*

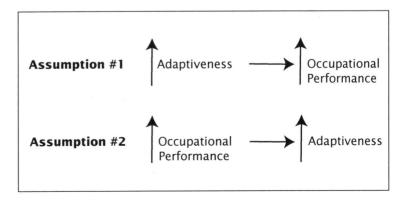

Figure 1. A comparison of underlying treatment assumptions.

Crist, P., & Royeen, C. (1997). Infusing Occupation into Practice. Bethesda, MD: American Occupational Therapy Association. *(This is a transcription of a workshop given by the theorists contrasting OA, MOHO, and Occupational Science using a mental health case example. Sally Schultz presents the OA perspective).*

Dolecheck, J. R., & Schkade, J. K. (1999) Effects on dynamic standing endurance when persons with CVA perform personally meaningful activities rather than non-meaningful tasks. *Occupational Therapy Journal of Research, 19*(1), 40–53. *(The patient case that inspired this study appears in the Christiansen & Baum book cited below [Schultz & Schkade, 1997.] It's a wonderful case!)*

Ford, K. (1995). Occupational adaptation in home health: A therapist's viewpoint. *Home Health and Community Special Interest Section Newsletter, American Occupational Therapy Association, 2*(1), 2–4. *(This is an excellent, easy-to-read article.)*

Garbarini, J., & Pearlman, V. (1998). Fieldwork in home health care: A model for practice. *Education Special Interest Section Quarterly, 8*(4), 1–4. *(This is an excellent example of use of OA to guide student practice in home health.)*

Garrett, S., & Schkade, J. K. (1995). The occupational adaptation model of professional development as applied to level II fieldwork in occupational therapy. *American Journal of Occupational Therapy, 49*, 119–126. *(This is a good explanation of the adaptive response behaviors.)*

Gibson, J., & Schkade, J. K. (1997). Effects of occupational adaptation treatment with CVA. *American Journal of Occupational Therapy, 51*, 523–529. *(This clinical study demonstrates functional outcomes.)*

Johnson, J., & Schkade, J. K. (in press). Effects of occupation-based intervention on mobility in CVA. *Journal of Applied Gerontology. (These three cases of home health intervention are excellent application examples.)*

Macrae, A., Falk-Dessler, J., Juline, D., Padilla, R., & Schultz, S. (1998). Occupational therapy models. In A. Macrae, & E. Cara (Eds.), *Psychosocial occupational therapy: A clinical practice* (pp. 97–125). Albany, NY: Delmar. *(This chapter describes the use of OA in mental health practice.)*

Pasek, P. B., & Schkade, J. K. (1996). Effects of a skiing experience on adolescents with limb deficiencies: An occupational adaptation perspective. *American Journal of Occupational Therapy, 50,* 24–31. *(The focus is on relative mastery construct.)*

Ross, M. M. (1994, August 11). Applying theory to practice. *OT Week,* 16–17. *(This nice case was written by a therapist who is an excellent practitioner of Occupational Adaptation).*

Schkade, J. K., & Schultz, S. (1992). Occupational adaptation: Toward a holistic approach to contemporary practice, Part 1. *American Journal of Occupational Therapy, 46,* 829–837. *(This is part one of an original article.)*

Schkade, J. K., & Schultz, S. (1993). Occupational adaptation: An integrative frame of reference in H. Hopkins, & H. Smith (Eds.). *Willard & Spackman's occupational therapy,* (8th ed.). Philadelphia: Lippincott. *(This is a brief description. The 1992 publication provides a more thorough understanding.)*

Schkade, J. K., & Schultz, S. (1993). Occupational adaptation: An example of theory and contemporary practice integration. Bethesda, MD: American Occupational Therapy Association, Commission on Education, Short Papers [Abstract].

Schkade, J. K., & Schultz, S. (1998). Occupational Adaptation: An integrative frame of reference in M.E. Neistadt & E.B. Crepeau (Eds.) *Willard & Spackman's occupational therapy* (9th ed.). Philadelphia: Lippincott. *(This is a short description, included with MOHO and Ecology of Human Performance as theories based on occupational behavior.)*

Schkade, J. K. (1999). Student to practitioner: The adaptive transition. *Innovations in Occupational Therapy Education,* 147–156. *(This has application to professional transitions.)*

Schultz, S., & Schkade, J. (1997). Adaptation in C. Christiansen & C. Baum, (Eds.). *Occupational therapy: Enabling function and well-being* (2nd ed.). Thorofare, N.J.: Slack, Inc. *(This is an extensive treatment of the concept of adaptation as a paradigm with a couple of cases using Occupational Adaptation. The theory is well articulated, and the most up-to-date definitions are included.)*

Schultz, S., & Schkade, J. K. (1992). Occupational adaptation: Toward a holistic approach to contemporary practice, Part 2. *American Journal of Occupational Therapy, 46,* 917–926. *(This is the second part of an original article).*

Schultz, S., & Schkade, J. K. (1994). Home health care: A window of opportunity to synthesize practice. *Home & Community Health, Special Interest Section Newsletter, American Occupational Therapy Association, 1*(3), 1–4. *(This is a good article for understanding the basic approach to intervention. We highly recommend this as a first article to read.)*

Manuscript submitted for publication

Jackson, J. P., & Schkade, J. K. (2000). Occupational adaptation model versus biomechanical/rehabilitation models in the treatment of patients with hip fractures.

Other recommended readings

On Challenge

Csikszentmihalyi, M. (1990). *Flow.* New York: Harper Collins Publishers.

On Transition

Dr. Seuss (1990). *Oh the places you'll go.* New York: Random House.

On a Balanced Lifestyle
(implications for adaptation energy)

McGee-Cooper, A. (1992). *You don't have to go home from work exhausted!* New York: Bantam.

On Adaptation

Johnson, S. (1998). *Who Moved My Cheese?* New York: Putnam.

Infusing Occupation Into Practice

Workshop sponsored by the Education Special Interest Section of the American Occupational Therapy Association at the 1999 Annual Conference and Exposition, April 16–20, 1999 in Indianapolis, Indiana.

Presenters

Ecology of Human Performance

Winnie Dunn, PhD, OTR, FAOTA

Professor and Chair, Department of Occupational Therapy Education, University of Kansas

Person-Environment Occupational Model

Mary Law, PhD, OT(C)

Associate Dean, Health Science (Rehabilitation); Director, School of Rehabilitation Science; and Co-Director, CanChild Centre For Childhood Disability Research

Conceptual Framework of Therapeutic Occupation (CFTO)

David Nelson, PhD, OTR, FAOTA

Professor, Department of Occupational Therapy Medical College of Ohio

Editors

Patricia A. Crist, PhD, OTR/L, FAOTA

Chair and Professor, Department of Occupational Therapy John G. Rangos, Sr. School of Health Sciences Duquesne University

Charlotte Brasic Royeen, PhD, OTR, FAOTA

Associate Dean for Research and Professor in Occupational Therapy, School of Pharmacy and Allied Health Professions, Creighton University

Janette K. Schkade, PhD, OTR, FAOTA

Professor and Dean, School of Occupational Therapy Texas Woman's University

Theoretical References

Ecology of Human Performance

Dunn, W., Brown, C. & McGuigan, A. (1994). The ecology of human performance: A framework for considering the effect of context. *American Journal of Occupational Therapy, 48*, 595–607.

Dunn, W., Brown, C., McClain, L., & Westman, K. (1994). The ecology of human performance: A contextual perspective on human occupation. In C. B. Royeen (Ed.) *AOTA self study series: The practice of the future: Putting occupation back into therapy,* Rockville, MD: American Occupational Therapy Association.

Person–Environment–Occupation Model

Law, M., Cooper, B., Strong, S, Stewart, D., Rigby, P. & Letts, L. (1996). The person-environment-occupation model: A transactive approach to occupational performance. *Canadian Journal of Occupational Therapy, 63*, 9–23.

Strong, S., Rigby, P., Stewart, D., Law, M., Letts, L. & Cooper, B. (in press). Application of the Person-Environment-Occupation model: A practical tool. *Canadian Journal of Occupational Therapy.*

Letts, L., Law, Rigby, P., Cooper, B., Stewart, D., & Strong, S. (1994). Person-environment assessments in occupational therapy. *American Journal of Occupational Therapy, 48*, 608–618.

Conceptual Framework of Therapeutic Occupation

Nelson, D. L (1998). Occupation: Form and performance. *American Journal of Occupational Therapy, 42,* 633–641.

Nelson, D. L. (1994). Occupational form, occupational performance, therapeutic occupation. In C. B. Royeen (Ed.) *AOTA self study series: The practice of the future: Putting occupation back into therapy, Lesson 2* (pp. 9–48). Rockville, MD: American Occupational Therapy Association.

Nelson, D. L. (1996). Therapeutic occupation: A definition. *American Journal of Occupational Therapy, 50,* 775–782.

Nelson, D. L. (1997). The 1996 Eleanor Clarke Slagle Lecture. Why the profession of occupational therapy will continue to flourish in the twenty-first century. *American Journal of Occupational Therapy, 51,* 11–24.

Introduction

Janette Schkade
Panel Moderator

Welcome to the American Occupational Therapy Association (AOTA) 1999 Annual Conference and Exposition, April 16–20, in Indianapolis, Indiana. We now join this session recorded live at the Indianapolis Convention Center. This session is the second in a series that began in Chicago at the Annual Conference in 1996. That event also made its way into the AOTA (1997) publication, *Infusing Occupation Into Practice,* which many of you, I hope, have been using. That monograph contains the proceedings from Chicago where three major approaches to occupation were compared across one common case study to demonstrate application of each approach during the occupational therapy intervention. The three approaches covered in the initial publication were Occupational Adaptation (Sally Schultz, PhD, OTR), Model of Human Occupation (Gary Kielhofner, DrPH, OTR/L) and Occupational Science (Florence Clark, PhD, OTR, FAOTA).

At the sesson in Indianapolis, our speakers were Winnie Dunn, Professor and Chair of the Department of Occupational Therapy at the University of Kansas Medical Center who discussed the Ecology of Human Performance; Mary Law, Professor, School of Rehabilitation Science, McMaster University in Canada presented the Person–Environment–Occupation Model; and David Nelson, Professor, Department of Occupational Therapy at the Medical College of Ohio, explained the benefits of the Conceptual Framework of Therapeutic Occupation.

Overview of Theoretical Models

Ecology of Human Performance

Winnie Dunn

The Ecology of Human Performance (EHP) is a framework that the University of Kansas designed for its graduate occupational therapy program. The faculty chose the word *ecology* very carefully. The definition of ecology is, "The totality of patterns of relationships between organisms and their environments" (Dunn, Brown, & McGuigan, 1994). We used the word *ecology* because we believed that this was exactly the essential feature of what occupational therapists need to think about; how organisms, in this case people, and their environments and the things and other people around them organize themselves to support or prohibit performance.

One of the core assumptions of the EHP is that people are embedded in their contexts, and to consider their performance without considering the context in which they must perform would be a misjudgment of their actual performance. The definition of context, according to AOTA (1994) *Uniform Terminology* includes temporal, physical, social, and cultural features. I think sometimes we think of a context as a physical environment or only a social environment, when, in fact, we also have temporal features, such as how far along persons are in their disability experience. Temporal context also includes what we expect of an 8-year-old compared with a 25-year-old. The differences may or may not be substantial. The issues of cultural context relate not only to ethnic issues, but also to the culture of a family and the expectations within the workplace. The social context relates expectations within the group of friends that you have.

So the first thing that we consider in this framework is what a person needs and wants to do. That sets the frame for us to consider the next things, such as where he or she is going to do it and how he or she is going to perform the desired task. Figure 2 is a schemata for the EHP (Dunn, Brown, & McGuigan, 1994).

The idea here is that the person is that small white figure embedded in the context. You cannot see the center (i.e., the person) until you get into the context because they are so meshed together. You can bite or lick or chew, but you have to take some action! So in the diagram, we have cut a little wedge out of the Tootsie Roll Pop so that we can see the center (i.e., the person), and that is our way

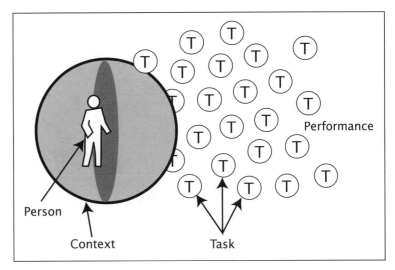

Figure 2. Schemata for the Ecology of Human Performance framework. Persons are imbedded in their contexts. An infinite variety of tasks exists around every person. Performance occurs as a result of the person interacting with context to engage in tasks. *Note.* From "The Ecology of Human Performance: A Framework for Considering the Effect of Context," p. 599, by W. Dunn, C. Brown, & A. McGuigan, 1994, *American Journal of Occupational Therapy, 48*, 595–607. Copyright 1994 by The American Occupational Therapy Association, Inc. Reprinted with permission.

of depicting that people are embedded in their contexts. The "Ts" on the outside represent tasks available in the universe. The idea is that tasks are universally available to everyone, and they are not inside the person or the context. They are just generic things that are available to everyone. When you look at the interaction then, people interact within their environments. You see this tootsie roll pop as a lens, the person interacts with the environment, and the interaction results in the performance range (see Figure 3). You see that some tasks come into range, and some tasks are outside of it because of the interaction between personal skills and the environmental variables that are available to the person. If you have fewer skills as an individual, you might be in the same environment as everybody else but you do not take advantage of those environmental variables because you do not have the skills, and, in that case your performance ranges become narrower. For example, a child with attention deficit hyperactivity disorder (ADHD) is in the same classroom with all the other children who know that when the teacher turns the lights off it is time to be quiet. The child with ADHD does not understand it; he has the same cue as everyone else, the same context as everyone else, but he does not have the skills inside of himself to recog-

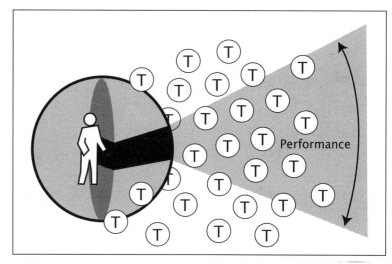

Figure 3. Schemata of a typical person within the Ecology of Human Performance framework. Persons use their skills and abilities to "look through" the context at the tasks they need or want to do. Persons derive meaning from this process. Performance range is the configuration of tasks that persons execute. *Note.* From "The Ecology of Human Performance: A Framework for Considering the Effect of Context," p. 600, by W. Dunn, C. Brown, & A. McGuigan, 1994, *American Journal of Occupational Therapy, 48,* 595–607. Copyright 1994 by The American Occupational Therapy Association, Inc. Reprinted with permission.

Winnie Dunn

nize the meaning of this particular event, so his performance range gets narrower (see Figure 4).

We can also have a situation in which the person has a certain number of skills but they are in an impoverished environment. I am a gourmet cook, and if I am in a cabin in the woods, it does not matter what gourmet cooking skills I have, my performance range is narrower because there are not the environmental supports for me to demonstrate those personal skills (see Figure 5).

I think the dilemma that occupational therapists sometimes face with people who have disabilities is the combination of an impoverished environment and impoverished personal skills, and that becomes a dilemma that all of us are challenged to address in our practice.

The EHP model has five interventions (see Figure 6):

1. *Establish/restore interventions, focus on person variables* means those restorative or remedial strategies that we have all learned.

2. *Adapt* (see the arrows pointing to task and context in Figure 6). The therapist knows what the person needs and wants to do, and you figure out a way for them to do it today. You make whatever

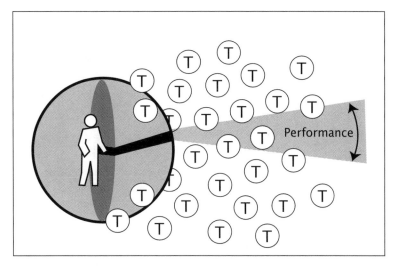

Figure 4. Schemata of a person with limited skills and abilities within the Ecology of Human Performance framework. Although context is still useful, the person has less skills and abilities to "look through" context and derive meaning. This limits the person's performance range. *Note.* From "The Ecology of Human Performance: A Framework for Considering the Effect of Context," p. 601, by W. Dunn, C. Brown, & A. McGuigan, 1994, *American Journal of Occupational Therapy, 48,* 595–607. Copyright 1994 by The American Occupational Therapy Association, Inc. Reprinted with permission.

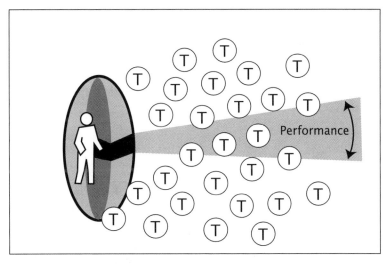

Figure 5. Schemata of a limited context within the Ecology of Human Performance framework. The person has adequate skills and abilities, but the context does not provide resources needed to perform. In this situation, performance range is limited. *Note.* From "The Ecology of Human Performance: A Framework for Considering the Effect of Context," p. 602, by W. Dunn, C. Brown, & A. McGuigan, 1994, *American Journal of Occupational Therapy, 48,* 595–607. Copyright 1994 by The American Occupational Therapy Association, Inc. Reprinted with permission.

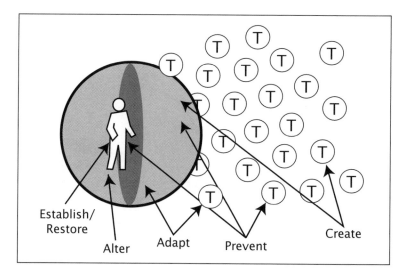

Establish/
Restore

Alter   Adapt   Prevent   Create

Figure 6. Illustration of therapeutic interventions within the Ecology of Human Performance framework. The arrows indicate the variables that are affected by each intervention. *Note.* From "The Ecology of Human Performance: A Framework for Considering the Effect of Context," p. 603, by W. Dunn, C. Brown, & A. McGuigan, 1994, *American Journal of Occupational Therapy, 48,* 595–607. Copyright 1994 by The American Occupational Therapy Association, Inc. Reprinted with permission.

Winnie Dunn

changes are necessary to the task or context variables for the person to have access to the activity. I think that is a hallmark of occupational therapy and a gift that we sometimes neglect to give in our attempt to always look at restoring and establishing skills. Sometimes we can give people the gift of doing right away by adapting things and providing immediate opportunity.

3. *Alter.* This intervention involves finding a better place. You do not ask the person to get better or the environment to change, you ask where is the best place for this person to enact his or her life.

We had a young man who had a head injury and he wanted to work. He had good social engagement skills but would get in others' personal space. He could enact the first social reciprocity behaviors, but then he would not leave their space. So his relationships always ended negatively with the other person saying, "Get away from me!" The question is do we put him in a social skills training program to see whether he deserves and can earn the right to work? No, we found him a job as a bagger at the grocery store. The customers loved him because he was so socially engaging with them and the counter acted as a barrier between them. He could not get in others' personal space, and the relationship ended positively when the customers finished checking out of the grocery store. At our grocery stores in Kansas City, we also drive up after the purchase and the baggers load our cars. So this young man got one more chance to engage with people but they were in their cars. He could load and talk and everyone thought he was a great bagger. We did not ask the grocery store to change, we did not ask him to get better before he earned the right to work, we just found a place that was a better match. That is a skill that occupational therapists can use, but frequently we neglect it. We always think that we have to keep fixing everything.

4. *Prevent* is an intervention in which you anticipate an outcome. The person is doing fine on the variable of interest, but he or she has the risk of getting worse. We do not wait until a person has decubitus ulcers to say, "Oh, I should have set up a positioning program." We do not wait for a third grader to act out in frustration with his peers before setting up some programs to increase positive socialization. Maybe we do sometimes, but we should not. Prevention is anticipation of an outcome and doing something now to change the course of that outcome in the interest of *growing* the person's skills.

5. *Create* is an intervention that I think in the next 10 to 15 years is going to be a critical feature of occupational therapy moving into the next phase of our evolution. We take our skills as a profession and apply them to the needs of a community in ways that are not about disability at all. When we serve on a park board, we help it to set up the parks so that everyone can play. We are not saying, "Tommy needs to play and we need to adapt the environment for Tommy." We say, "This is in the best interest of everyone." I think the best example of this is the Americans With Disabilities Act of 1990, which requires us to have curb cuts. Do you know who the Number 1 user of curb cuts is? Parents with strollers, not persons with disabilities. I think knowledge and expertise in occupational therapy can be used in the interest of living a quality life that has nothing to do with whether you have a disability and has everything to do with whether your life is satisfying and available to you. So I think that is an important intervention for us to consider as we move into the next decade where funding and other resources are changing, providing us with the opportunity to be where we should have been in the first place.

Person–Environment–Occupation Model

Mary Law

The Person–Environment–Occupational (PEO) Model was developed with a number of colleagues at McMaster University in Canada over the past 9 years (Law et al., 1996). We shared an interest in

Mary Law   occupation-based practice as well as an interest in environmental issues—both theory and research. Additionally, we had a sense that intervention focused on the environment, and environmental issues could be much more powerful than some of the interventions that we normally do.

The PEO Model has theoretical foundations that come from the *Occupational Therapy Guidelines for Client-Centered Practice* (Canadian Association of Occupational Therapists [CAOT], 1997). These are Canadian guidelines that have been around since the early 1980s and were recently updated in 1997. The Model is also based on environmental theories developed by Lawton and Brofenbrenner as well as the theory of optimal experience or flow (Bronfenbrenner, 1997; Lawton, 1986). The expected outcome of this theoretical model is an improved fit among person, occupation, and environment. We theorize that the improved fit will result in optimal occupational performance. Figure 7 shows how we depict our model graphically. It shows that occupational performance results from a dynamic transactive relationship among person, occupation, and environment.

We define person as a human being who assumes different roles and presents a balance of mind, body, and spiritual characteristics. People possess both attributes and skills, which they contribute to their everyday life. Environment is defined very broadly as physi-

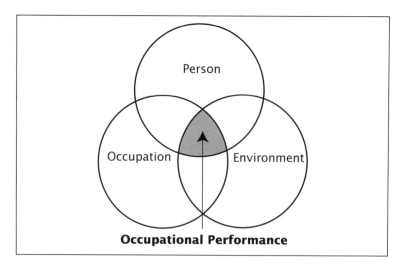

Figure 7. Person-Environment-Occupation Model of Occupational Performance. From "The Person-Environment-Occupation Model: A Transactive Approach to Occupational Performance," by M. Law, B. Cooper, S. Strong, D. Stewart, P. Rigby, & L. Letts, 1996, *Canadian Journal of Occupational Therapy, 63(1)*, p. 9–23. Copyright 1996 by the Canadian Association of Occupational Therapists. Reprinted with permission.

cal, social, cultural, and institutional, and ranges from the person to his or her family, neighborhood, community, province or state, country, and world. Occupation is defined as groups of self-directed tasks or activities in which we engage over a lifespan. Occupational performance results from the dynamic experience of when we engage in purposeful activities and tasks within our environment. So there is really a large emphasis on the person's subjective experience of doing occupations in the PEO Model.

We have a number of assumptions within the PEO Model about occupational performance. It is complex and dynamic and has both temporal and spatial considerations. It changes across time and across space. Too often, we look at persons as one slice in time without looking at what has happened in their occupational profile and what can be projected into the future.

Occupational performance is shaped by the transaction among person, environment, and occupation. It changes over our lifetimes. It changes as we change our priorities in terms of what we want or need to do. Occupational performance requires a balance, but this is an individualized balance. There is no balance that is prescriptive or best for each person. It has some observable qualities that you can measure objectively, but, primarily, it is a subjective experience and is best measured by self-report.

One of the primary uses of the PEO Model is as an analytic tool so that you can look at how changes in person, environment, or occupation can either maximize or minimize the fit. If there is increased fit among person, environment, and occupation, then you will have more optimal occupational performance. You can analyze what is happening in terms of the person at this point in time, what has happened in the past, and what you can project will happen in the future.

The major assumptions of the PEO Model are that these components (person, environment, occupation) interact continually over time and space, resulting in a relationship that can vary in terms of the congruence of the fit. Optimal occupational performance occurs with the best fit. This is not necessarily due to all three coming together, but it could be one overlapping much more than the other.

Figure 8 depicts the influence of person, environment, and occupation over a lifespan. As you can see, there are many times in our lives, even times within each day, when we have optimal fit and optimal occupational performance.

Acknowledgment

I wish to thank fellow members of the Environmental Research Group at McMaster University—Barbara Cooper, Lori Letts, Debra Stewart, Susan Strong and Patti Rigby (University of Toronto).

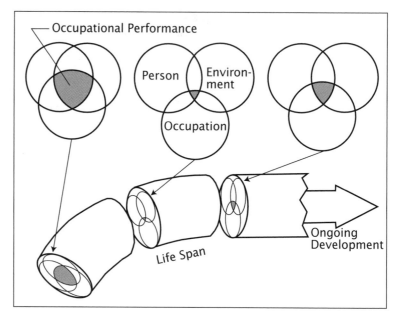

Figure 8. The Transactional Relationship Between Person, Their Environments and Occupation Over a Lifespan. From "The Person-Environment-Occupation Model: A Transactive Approach to Occupational Performance," by M. Law, B. Cooper, S. Strong, D. Stewart, P. Rigby, & L. Letts, 1996, *Canadian Journal of Occupational Therapy, 63(1)*, p. 9–23. Copyright 1996 by the Canadian Association of Occupational Therapists. Reprinted with permission.

Conceptual Framework of Therapeutic Occupation

David Nelson

The Conceptual Framework of Therapeutic Occupation provides definitions of occupational concepts and specifies the relationships among these concepts (Nelson, 1988). At the Medical College of Ohio, we call this framework CFTO. Figure 9 is a diagram of CFTO's definition of occupation. Following is a list of basic definitions that you might find helpful:

■ *Occupational form:* the objective set of circumstances, external to the person, that elicits, guides, or structures the person's occupational performance.

■ *Occupational performance:* the voluntary doing of the person in the context of the occupational form.

■ *Meaning:* the entire interpretive process in which a person engages when encountering an occupational form.

■ *Purpose:* the experience of wanting an outcome to result from occupational performance. Purpose is the link between meaning, developmental structure, and occupational performance.

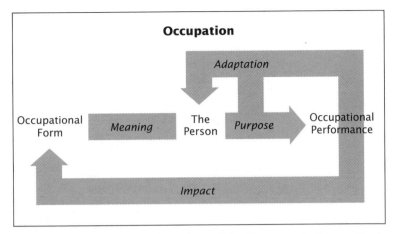

Figure 9. The Conceptual Framework for Therapeutic Occupation's (CFTO) definition of occupation. *Note.* From "Why the Profession of Occupational Therapy Will Flourish in the 21st Century, 1996 Eleanor Clarke Slagle Lecture," p. 13, by D. L. Nelson, 1997, *American Journal of Occupational Therapy, 51*, 11–24. Copyright 1997 by The American Occupational Therapy Association, Inc. Reprinted with permission.

- *Impact:* the effect of occupational performance on the subsequent occupational form.

- *Occupational adaptation:* the effect of a person's purpose and occupational performance on his or her developmental structure.

- *Occupational compensation:* Compensation involves a somewhat atypical occupational form, a substitute occupational performance, and an impact comparable to the impact of naturalistic occupational performance.

I would like to explain CFTO by getting right into the case. Ms. Irene Miller, according to the case description, is of Eastern European heritage, which gives us some information, but to understand the occupational form fully from a cultural point of view, we need specific detail. In occupational therapy, the particulars of occupational existence are everything. To give the case specificity of detail, I enlisted the help of the Medical College of Ohio Pi Theta Epsilon students. We made the assumptions that Ms. Miller is of Hungarian extraction and that she has lived all her life in a Hungarian neighborhood in Toledo. Figure 10 presents a map of the parts of the city that are most relevant. The coded house is her neighborhood; the Budapest Restaurant is in the west; the Toledo Storms play hockey, one of her favorite occupations to observe, near the Maumee River; and St. Charles Hospital, where she underwent acute care hospitalization, is in the lower right. St. Charles Hospital is a long way from home. The neighborhood hospital closer to home in

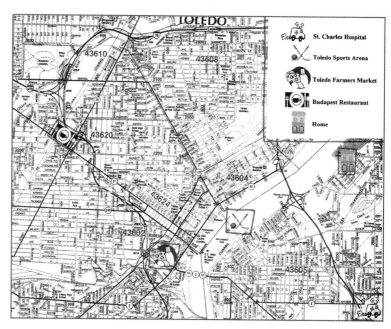

Figure 10. Simulation: Map of parts of the city that are meaningful to this particular person.

David Nelson   the Hungarian neighborhood (where her husband died) is closed. From now on, I am going to refer to Ms. Irene Miller as Irene because, in our scenario, that is the way she wants to be called.

Let's begin to explain CFTO by analyzing Irene's occupation at the personal care home described in the case description sent to us. Irene's occupational form (as we imagine it, in the personal care home) is characterized by standardized well-regulated care, with a special emphasis on safety. The personal care home is her world; it is a total institution. One problem of this world is the cultural and behavioral diversity of residents and staff. She is not familiar with the culture of the staff, or with the behavioral patterns of those who are designated her peers. Most residents have progressive dementia, but she has traumatic brain injury—a very different pattern of disorder. Television, group crafts, and exercise groups characterize the daily regimen of the personal care home. Two specific examples of routine occurrences in her occupational form include (a) the dinnertime use of cheap silverware that Irene would never use for company in her own house and (b) the tendency for staff to dress up older ladies in clothes that are functional but atypical of what most older women wear in public settings.

If, in general, this is a description of her occupational form, then, in general, what is her occupational performance? Occupational performance is the objectively observable, voluntary doing of the person in the context of the occupational form. In the case of Irene, let us posit that there is verbal and nonverbal complaining about staff, roommates, other residents, and facilities. There are periods of agitation alternating with passive tearfulness. On the positive side, there is regular participation in Catholic religious services. During family visits, Irene varies between cheerful compliance and desperate pleas. She says, "I don't want to die here." Irene's occupational performance is shaped and limited by her occupational form.

Form and performance are objectively observable, but in CFTO's definition of occupation, subjective experience is also essential. So let us consider her felt and personal meanings. Some of the meanings she experiences in the context of occupational form include (a) fears of increased disability and death, (b) painful awareness of decreased memory and problem-solving ability, (c) frustration with immobility and pain, (d) boredom, (e) loneliness and felt aloofness from other residents, and (f) deep religiosity and hope. These meanings are powerful to her; they arise and evolve as she encounters her occupational form on a daily basis.

In CFTO, once meaning is established, purpose follows. What are Irene's purposes? What does she want? What is her goal orientation, her heartfelt desire? In summary, let us assume that (a) she has deep desires to escape, to go home, and, in general, to live; (b) she wants things to return to the way they were before the accident; (c) she has a vague desire to be polite and to comply with the demands of others; and (d) she has a minimal desire to participate in the daily routine of enforced self-care and passive recreation.

Having introduced Irene's occupational form, occupational performance, meanings, and purposes, we now note that the definition of occupation also involves the dynamics of occupation over time. The dynamics of occupation include impact and adaptation. Impact is the effect of occupational performance on subsequent occupational forms (it is the effect one has on one's world). In contrast, adaptation is the change in one's own person because of active occupational performance.

What are Irene's impacts in the personal care home? Little! She cannot go where she wants (she cannot change her surroundings). She cannot do things for her son and grandchildren. She has trivial impacts only.

So, what are her adaptations? She has adapted to her occupational form (the personal care home) with (a) an increased fear of death and disability, (b) a decreased belief in her own capacities, (c) an increased distrust of others, (d) reinforcement of maladaptive patterns of movement, and (e) reinforcement of maladaptive cognitive patterns and preoccupations. In summary, her occupation in the setting has led to maladaptation.

David Nelson   We have posited Irene's occupational patterns in the personal care home through the use of CFTO. Now it is important to point out that CFTO is a broad conceptual framework, not a model of practice (frame of reference). CFTO is compatible with all the different occupational therapy models of practice, but by design, it does not provide practical guidelines for intervention, as does a model of practice. So we need to select a model of practice in the case of Irene. In CFTO, the definition of a truly occupational model of practice has two main parts: (a) There is a theory of healthy occupation and threats to occupation, and (b) there are practical guidelines for synthesizing therapeutic occupational forms, for evaluation as well as intervention. Every occupational therapy model of practice has these basic characteristics, and the therapist who uses CFTO must select a model of practice providing these theory-based yet practical guidelines for intervention through occupation.

The model of practice to be used today for the case of Irene has been developed by a colleague of mine at the Medical College of Ohio, Lynne Chapman, MS, OTR. We can call her model an emerging model of practice (Chapman, 1996). The special focus of Chapman's model of practice consists of the occupational problems typically experienced by a person with traumatic brain injury. This model draws from and integrates principles of (a) community-based practice, (b) therapeutic community, (c) contemporary cognitive intervention, and (d) and neurodevelopmental treatment. I will try to show how CFTO can be integrated with Chapman's model of practice to guide occupational therapy intervention in the posited case of Irene.

Acknowledgments

I thank Lynne Chapman, MS, OTR; the members of the Alpha Omicron Chapter of Pi Theta Epsilon; Martin Rice, PhD, OTR; and Lisa Link Melville, MS, OTR.

Case Study:
Long Journey Home

This case by Linda Dunal, BSc, OT(c), is published in the *Canadian Occupational Therapy Foundation Case Study Review—Outcomes That Matter in Occupational Therapy,* p. 44, by the Canadian Occupational Therapy Foundation, 1998. ©1998 by the Canadian Occupational Therapy Foundation. Adapted with permission.

The case has been modified for the purposes of the Education Special Interest Section Workshop, *Infusing Occupation Into Practice II—A Comparative Case Study of Three Approaches,* American Occupational Therapy Association 1999 Annual Conference and Exposition, Saturday, April 17, 1999, Indianapolis, Indiana.

Case History

Ms. Irene Miller is a 70-year-old widow who as led a very active life. She walked 2 to 3 miles a day through her lifelong neighborhood replete with familiar Eastern European culture and customs. She was a volunteer at the local public library and an avid reader. She regularly attended her community church activities. In August 1997, Irene was hit by a car during one of her daily outings and suffered a closed head injury. Her computed tomography scan showed a small parietal acute subdural hematoma and large frontal temporal contusions. Although she initially received inpatient rehabilitation, she became confused and agitated and was admitted to a behavior management unit in late 1997. By the summer of 1998, she was walking with a walker and one-person assistance; needing assistance in a wheelchair for long distances; and requiring maximum assistance for all activities of daily living, although she was able to feed herself if her tray was set up. Irene's biggest challenges were her poor memory and difficulty with problem solving and communication, which was limited to the occasional sentence or question with the tendency to repeat syllables as she became excited. She had and still does have a supportive son who lives in the community. She currently resides in a personal care home close to the hospital. A caregiver arranged by her case manager assists her 2 hours a day with self-tasks. By November 1998, Irene's physical and cognitive status were stabilized, and her son wanted to see whether she could live at home with a live-in caregiver. Irene was also interested in returning home. She missed visiting her friends, going to church, reading children's stories at the library, browsing new and old bookstores, and being able to prepare foods she liked.

Current Clinical Considerations

Irene can sit unsupported for a few minutes. She was able to manage a one-person standing pivot transfer, but became quite anxious on any movement. She was not able to consistently and independently propel the wheelchair. A home visit was carried out with Irene and her son. She seemed to be aware that she was home. Irene lived in a two-story townhouse with an 8-inch, one-step entrance. On the main floor were a powder room, kitchen, and an open dining and living room combination. Irene's son was able to tilt her wheelchair up the front entrance step easily. The main floor doorways were all wide enough to accommodate the wheelchair except for the powder room. A straight flight of stairs lead up to the second floor bedroom. Irene could manage the stair with two persons assisting but was quite frightened, and it took a lot of encouragement to get her down safely. Once upstairs, she could hold onto the railing and walk to her bedroom with one person assisting. She needed help to get on and off the toilet. She could not get into the bathtub or shower.

At this time, the occupational therapy practitioner was aware that Irene had been depressed about her current living, health, and activity quality of life. She frequently is tearful over this desire. Irene was not going to be an independent propeller. Although she is able to communicate more clearly, she was only able to use simple sentences or questions. She continues to have poor memory and difficulty with problem solving.

Case Study Questions

1. On the basis of your theoretical reference, how do you begin to understand this person? How do you assess and evaluate or understand function and dysfunction (*initial assessment*)?

2. On the basis of your theoretical reference, how would you begin the intervention process? Or, how would factors influencing the unfolding of the person's story be considered (*intervention process*)?

3. On the basis of your theoretical reference, what are projected outcomes for this person (*intervention outcomes*)?

4. What future research questions are viable or needed to study clinical application of your work (*future clinical research*)?

Case Study Discussion

Initial Assessment

On the basis of your theoretical reference, how would you begin the intervention process? How do you assess and evaluate or understand function and dysfunction?

Winnie Dunn
Ecology of Human Performance

From an Ecology of Human Performance (EHP) perspective, we begin by asking: "What does Irene want and need to do?" Our case study material informs us that she wants to return home and reconnect with activities such as volunteering, cooking, and spending time with friends. Secondly, we determine where (i.e., context) the person needs and wants to perform. For Irene, her wish is to live in her neighborhood community.

The assessment would begin with interviews and skilled observation of Irene as she tries daily life and other desired tasks. We would also begin gathering information about her home, neighborhood, support systems, etc. We also have a lot of information about Irene's status. For example, she has low endurance, poor memory skills, and hemiparesis. We see these person–variable features as we observe Irene; we can also see how these person–variable challenges are affecting her performance.

We will consider what Irene wants and needs to do, where she will do these tasks, and what supports and barriers we see in her performance as we interpret the data and begin to plan our intervention options with Irene.

Mary Law
Person–Environment–Occupation Model

Using the Person–Environment–Occupation (PEO) Model, we would begin the intervention process with an interview with Irene to enable her to identify the occupational performance issues that are currently important to her. We believe that function and dysfunction are best understood by hearing from the person herself, what she wants to be able to do, needs to do, or is expected to do. The outcome measure that we feel is best suited to this identification process is the Canadian Occupational Performance Measure (COPM) (Law et al., 1998). The COPM is useful in a situation such as Irene's because it enables her to identify her major performance issue, which is returning home, along with the other activities that she wants or needs to be able to do when she does return home.

Through the initial interview, we will learn the issues that are important to Irene. The same process can be used with her son to identify issues that are important to him regarding his mother. It is clear from the interview that Irene is a person with an independent and spiritual nature who has set clear goals for herself. In the past, she enjoyed a wide diversity of occupations, was independent in daily and community living skills, and enjoyed regular social occasions with her friends. She lives in a close-knit neighborhood with her son nearby and has a well-developed social network. We would look at her experience of occupations as of November 1998. As David has discussed, it is a very restrictive experience.

Once Irene has identified the occupational performance issues that are important to her, the occupational therapist, together with Irene and her family, would continue evaluation focused on the performance components and environmental conditions that sup-

Mary Law

port or hinder her current performance of identified activities. For example, her primary identified issue is to return to the home. The activities that she wants to be able to do to return home include moving around her home, completing basic self-care activities and helping with meal preparation. An assessment of performance components and environmental conditions would be completed in relation to the specific activities. Evaluation of components not required for these activities is unnecessary. Other assessments that could be used in this process include the Enabler-R (Iwarsson & Isacsson, 1996) and the Safety Assessment of Function (Letts, Scott, Burtney, Marshall, & McKean, 1998) and the Kitchen Task Assessment (Baum & Edwards, 1994). Both assessments look at functional activities in relationship to the home environment. The SAFER looks specifically at safety issues in the home. The Kitchen Task Assessment could be used to assess Irene's ability to assist in meal preparation. The advantage of this assessment is that it also provides information about performance components that either support or interfere with this activity.

The evaluation process developed for use in the PEO Model is not meant to be lengthy and if focused on the activities important to the client, can be completed in one or two therapy sessions. Results of this evaluation process for Irene provide us with the following issues and information that have an impact on Irene's person, environment, and occupation (See Table 1).

We tend to forget the tremendous influence we have in how evaluation and intervention proceeds. In this model, we stress the environment. In terms of evaluation of the environment for Irene, we would look at the physical, sociocultural, institutional and economic aspects of her environment in terms of whether she has the resources to go home. From a physical and economic point of view, what sorts of services are available? What are her son's expectations and what support is available from her social network?

The information gathered through the evaluation process would be brought together by the therapist, Irene, and her son to develop an intervention plan. The goal of intervention is to improve Irene's occupational performance in the activities that she has identified as important to her.

David Nelson
Conceptual Framework
of Therapeutic
Occupation

Figure 11 depicts the evaluation process from the Conceptual Framework of Therapeutic Occupation (CFTO) point of view (Nelson, 1994; Nelson, 1996).

In occupational assessment, the therapist collaboratively synthesizes occupational forms that are meaningful and purposeful to

Table 1. Results of the Evaluation Process of the PEO Model

Personal Impact of Disability
    Independent spirit
        Emotional status
        Mobility
        Memory
        Problem solving
        Communication

Experience of Occupation
    Restricted occupational profile
      Self-care
        Household mobility
      Productivity
        Transportation
        Volunteer work
      Leisure
        Reading
        Church activities

Environmental Influences
    Physical
      Accessibility of home and community
      Resources available
    Sociocultural
      Son's expectations and experiences
      Social network
    Institutional
      Service availability
      Service providers
      Economic

the person. The therapist observes the person's occupational performance in the context of the occupational form (assessment data), and makes inferences about his or her developmental structure.

As we use Chapman's (1996) emerging model of practice, to begin the assessment process from a CFTO point of view, we must make some assumptions. Our first assumption is that Irene has been referred to a community-based occupational therapist to help in the transition from the personal-care home to her own home in Toledo, Ohio. Our second assumption deals with funding. The reality is that

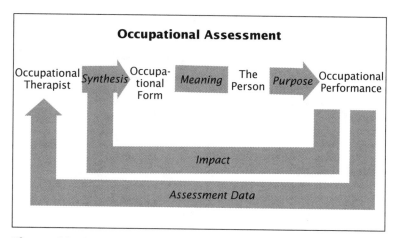

Figure 11. CFTO's depiction of the evaluation process.

David Nelson

a model of practice must consider funding. In Irene's case, we assume that the insurance company of the driver who injured Irene is responsible for her rehabilitation. The unfortunate fact of our times is that it would be necessary to scale back therapy if Irene had to rely on Medicare only.

The occupational therapist recognizes the importance of Irene's neighborhood and home as her future occupational form. So the evaluation starts in the neighborhood, which is a reflection of her culture. The therapist wants to observe Irene's occupational performance in her naturalistic occupational form and wants to make inferences about the match between form and performance so that therapeutic goals can be established. Later, the therapist will conduct formal assessments of cognition and motor ability at the clinic, but the most important part of the evaluation process is the observation of Irene in naturalistic settings.

Here is a map of her neighborhood (see Figure 12). I advocate the use of maps in beginning to understand the actual circumstances of peoples' lives. In the map, you see her home at the top, and the second most important place for Irene is St. Stephen's Church (indicated by the steeple). St. Stephen is the patron saint of Hungary, and the statue of St. Stephen outside the church has profound meaning to Irene. Our patients do not expect us to know everything about their cultures, but a good therapist is open to cues that clients provide about their cultures. Back to the map, there is the library where she used to volunteer, according to the case description. These are the actual locations in Toledo of the library and the church. On the map you see Magyar Street, which demonstrates the Hungarian influence, and the world-famous Tony Packo's restaurant. Tony Packo's restaurant is where *M*A*S*H*'s Corporal

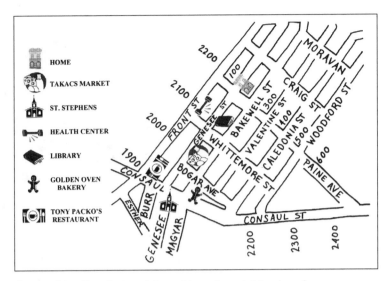

Figure 12. Simulation: Map of Irene's neighborhood.

Klinger wanted to return to from the war in Korea; the actor Jamie Farr is actually from this neighborhood and incorporated it into the TV show. To give you more of a flavor of the neighborhood, Figure 13 is a photograph of Takac's Meats with the Hungarian flag on the store. But note the problem that the concrete step will pose for Irene in her wheelchair. She will also have trouble seeing the tops of the counters in this colorful, but inaccessible store. Figure 14 shows Haas's Hungarian, Polish, and American pastries and baked goods, and Figure 15 shows the Hungarian club where Irene has socialized for much of her life.

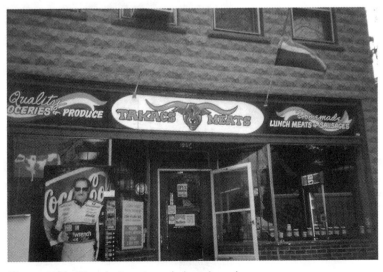

Figure 13. Simulation: Irene's butcher shop.

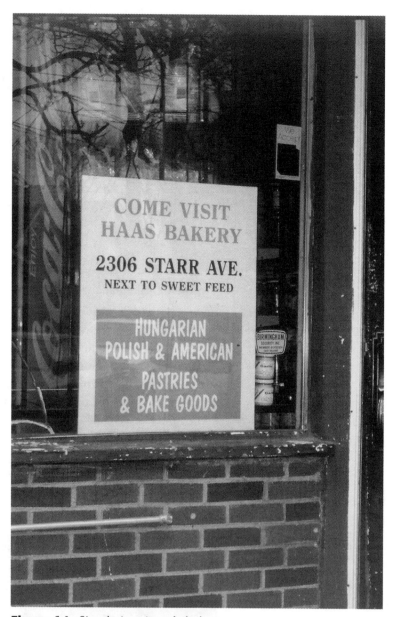

Figure 14. Simulation: Irene's bakery.

David Nelson

Figure 16 is a photograph of Tony Packo's restaurant, where Irene has enjoyed going to listen to the band on Saturday nights. She likes the chicken pakrikash. The occupational therapist notices the nice wheelchair access to the main part of the restaurant. However, there are four steps up to the only women's restroom, and the therapist realizes that much planning will be necessary for Irene to negotiate those steps. We are meeting Irene's son at Tony Packo's. We had a lot of fun making these maps and photos of typical scenes in a Toledo neighborhood, and I hope you appreciate them, but of course,

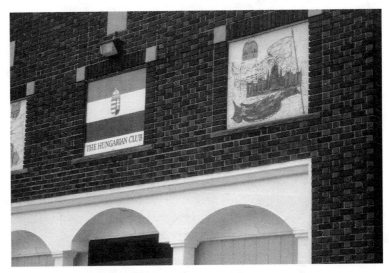

Figure 15. Simulation: Irene's social club.

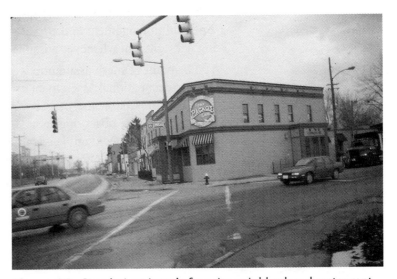

Figure 16. Simulation: Irene's favorite neighborhood restaurant.

the main point is that CFTO requires specificity in the description
of occupational forms and occupational performances.

In our posited evaluation process, the occupational therapist notes
Irene's son's devotion to helping his mother but the therapist is
initially puzzled by Irene's reticence to allow him to supervise her
money management. This creates a problem because of Irene's need
for assistance in this area. Only over time does Irene reveal to the
occupational therapist that her son is recovering from a gambling
problem. So Irene and the occupational therapist work out a plan
for her cousin to take care of finances. The point here is that a

David Nelson

community-based model of practice deals with unique family situations, not with stereotypical roles. Evaluation is a gradual process in which the situation is revealed to the therapist after a successful history of collaborative problem-solving has been built up.

We said that cognitive theories also influence Chapman's (1996) model of practice. Through observation of Irene in a naturalistic occupational form—Irene's neighborhood—the occupational therapist realizes that Irene has decreased contextual memory with inattention to relevant detail. Irene has problems with problem solving, especially in unanticipated situations. Her occasional agitation has different levels from mild nervousness to physical expression, and it is triggered by sensory overload and apparently insoluble problems in the occupational form.

We also said that neurodevelopmental treatment is a factor in Chapman's model. In the sensorimotor area, the therapist observes that Irene has right hemiparesis with increased tone of the right upper extremity and right lower extremity. She is currently experiencing a painful impingement in the right shoulder, and she avoids moving her right arm whenever possible.

The point of these assumptions is to communicate that CFTO depicts occupational assessment as the synthesis of occupational forms. In this case, the neighborhood outing with Irene is the synthesis. While observing Irene's occupational performance in settings that are meaningful and purposeful to her, the therapist can draw inferences about her developmental structure and occupational configuration. As with Irene, we always discover that each person's occupational reality, objective and subjective, is rich, surprising, and unique.

Intervention Process

On the basis of your theoretical reference, how would you begin the intervention process? Or, how would factors influencing the unfolding of the person's story be considered?

Winnie Dunn
Ecology of Human
Performance

The intervention process from an EHP perspective would cause us to look at sort of a parallel play activity. In other words, we would address some of the things that Irene is wanting to do in the personal care home as part of her recapturing a sense of herself and her sense of having some competence at doing the things she wants to do, and, simultaneously, we would plan with community care workers, the friends, and the social workers to try to make a plan about this new living situation. Irene does not need to just sit at the personal care home while we all make the big plan of how we are going to transition her to the community. She needs to feel as though she is developing a sense of recapturing her life. So while in the personal care home, she wants to be with her friends, she wants to do some of the church-gathering activities, and she wants to read with children at the library. She likes touring or visiting bookstores and she likes to cook. From an EHP perspective, we would look at all the different ways in which we can construct those activities in the personal care home. Sometimes there is a rolling cart with a library that Irene could visit. We could make arrangements with the care team to have the mobile library visit the care home. We could get some ideas about the kind of books she likes to read. Her son could bring some books from her personal library that she could just set around to create a context that supports her return to that identity. We could also set up visits for preschool children, day-care programs, or Girl Scout troops (or whatever is in her neighborhood) to come to the personal care home, and she could do activities with them such as reading or coloring or looking at books similar to whatever she did at the library to help her reconnect with the volunteer aspect of her identity.

From an EHP perspective we would do this simultaneously while planning with the team about what the personal living situation will be when she leaves. I think that from an intervention perspective, that part of the intervention planning would be related to looking at her finances and other personal resources. Does she have insurance or personal resources to have her house adapted so that she can get up and down the stairs and so that she can get to places in her home safely? Some people do. Perhaps she can get a stairglider to get up the stairs to get to her bedroom, which would be great. If she does not have those resources, then the team would look at other alternatives.

From an EHP perspective, we would look at all the alternatives regardless of resources, so that the family might have time to think about what they want to do. We would look at first floor apartments or condominiums or things that are in that neighborhood so that she would still feel a sense of place.

My mother has a lot of wisdom that she shares. One of the things she always say to me is, "Winnie, home is where your stuff is." That sense of agitation that Irene might have about change might be minimized by planning to get her stuff in these other places. We might take some of Irene's things to the places she visits so that she will have a sense of her own place before she makes choices about living there.

Winnie Dunn   Another thing that I thought of related to intervention planning and the finance issues is that if this is an old family home and she does not want to detach from that, the team and family might find a way for someone to rent it so that she would have an income while she lived in a different place but still feel a sense of owning the family home and having it as part of her life.

The other intervention thing would be to start working on planning for a personal care provider to come into the home because it is clear from the endurance issues that Irene would need to have people with her during the day. The team would try to set up some options to help the son and Irene negotiate how they are going to get this support. My mother just had knee surgery this week so siblings are taking turns taking care of her. She started crying with me a few weeks ago. She said "Winnie, I just don't want people in my home all the time. I lived alone for a long time." I think that sometimes we don't think about that. Sometimes we think about the care. If we do not think about things from a context perspective, we think about the person being cared for. Maybe they just need to be quiet and be alone and not feel as though they have to talk to somebody or behave a certain way. Mom says, "If I want to scream and cry, I want to scream and cry and I don't want someone to say 'Mary, it will be alright.'" So I think that we have to think about those kinds of things with Irene as well.

Mary Law
Person–Environment–
Occupational Model

In terms of intervention, where would I begin? I totally agree with what Dr. Dunn said that you start now and look at what can be done while she is still in the personal-care home. So I would begin with the client's goals. I made some assumptions about what the goals might be that she would identify on the COPM. These are:

- Move around my home
- Do some basic self-care, such as toileting
- Help prepare meals because I enjoy cooking
- Participate in activities at my church and the library
- See my friends

The intervention assumptions that I made are that she will return to live at home and that her performance components are stable.

To begin intervention, I would start with analysis of the interacting factors that affect performance (e.g., see Figure 17). I would look at person–occupation, occupation–environment, and person–environment. In terms of person–occupation, I would look at her skills and abilities and whether they match the requirements of the task, her perception of control and autonomy, and the value of

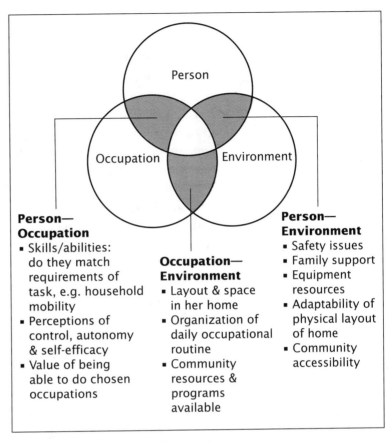

Person—
Occupation
- Skills/abilities:
  do they match
  requirements of
  task, e.g. household
  mobility
- Perceptions of
  control, autonomy
  & self-efficacy
- Value of being
  able to do chosen
  occupations

Occupation—
Environment
- Layout & space
  in her home
- Organization of
  daily occupational
  routine
- Community
  resources &
  programs
  available

Person—
Environment
- Safety issues
- Family support
- Equipment
  resources
- Adaptability of
  physical layout
  of home
- Community
  accessibility

Figure 17. Factors that affect performance.

being able to choose her own occupations. In terms of occupation–environment, I would look at the lay out and space in her home, organization of her daily occupational routine, and what community resources are available. In terms of person–environment, there are issues related to safety, family support, equipment resources, and adaptability of the physical layout of her home and community accessibility. I would use this to work together with Irene and her son to choose the initial focus of intervention.

So where are we going to get the "biggest bang for our buck?" In my opinion, that would occur by focusing on occupation and environment. Note that there is no intervention focused on the person. In terms of occupation, we would look at altering task demands and establishing a daily occupational routine that was satisfying to her. The major focus would be on the environment, both within the home and the community. We would look at issues relating to accessibility, program availability, and equipment. For example, I would start by seeing whether we could rent some equipment to do a trial stay in the home and see how that would work.

David Nelson
Conceptual Framework
for Therapeutic
Occupation

Because of time limitations, I am going to discuss occupational compensation as an intervention in this section, and I will discuss occupational adaptation in my answer to Question 3. Figure 18 is a diagrammatic depiction of occupational compensation.

In CFTO, occupational compensation involves a somewhat atypical occupational form, a substitute occupational performance, and a comparable impact (Nelson, 1994; Nelson 1996). Given her current motoric and cognitive abilities, how can Irene live at home? Given her current motoric and cognitive abilities how can Irene engage in desired occupations outside of the home?

A specific example of occupational compensation can be seen in the context of Irene's entry into St. Stephen's Church, which is so important to her. Figure 19 is a photo of the back door of St. Stephen's Church, which is a grand old church built in the 1920s with inaccessible front steps. A wheelchair lift is on the side of those steps. The somewhat artificial occupational form is the wheelchair lift (it is not the typical way for most people to get up the steps). The substitute occupational performance on Irene's part is sitting erect in the chair as the lift rises (this substitutes walking up the steps). The comparable impact is that Irene gets to the top of the stairs (she has a new occupational form, enabling entry into the church).

The occupational therapist in our scenario found that the wheelchair lift was in a state of disrepair. The men's club of the church mobilized themselves to fix it for Irene's benefit. More importantly, St. Stephen's community took it upon themselves to take turns in getting Irene to daily Mass every day at 7:15 a.m. This is an example of how the occupational therapist can be aided by community

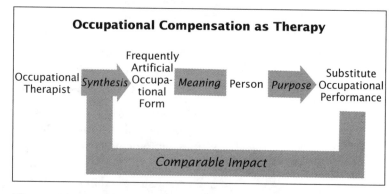

Figure 18. CFTO's depiction of occupational compensation. *Note.* From "Why the Profession of Occupational Therapy Will Flourish in the 21st Century, 1996 Eleanor Clarke Slagle Lecture," p. 15, by D. L. Nelson, 1997, *American Journal of Occupational Therapy, 51,* 11–24. Copyright 1997 by The American Occupational Therapy Association, Inc. Reprinted with permission.

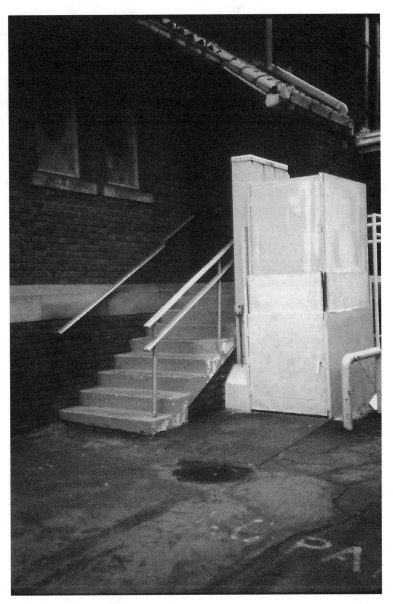

Figure 19. Simulation: Wheelchair lift at rear of Irene's place of worship.

resources; it is important for the community-based therapist to be alert to these kinds of resources.

In Irene's home are many doilies and afghans. She also has throw rugs and soft chairs and sofas out of which no person comes easily, especially Irene (Figure 20). The occupational therapist wins the family's confidence as she recommends compensatory changes and assistive devices for use in the home. Both safety and full participation in occupational life are stressed. These changes and devices can

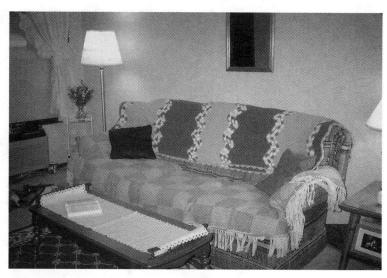

Figure 20. Simulation: Irene's living room.

David Nelson

be thought of as somewhat artificial occupational forms that have meaning and purpose to the individual. The occupational therapist explains occupational therapy as she makes her recommendations. A critical part of that explanation is a clear definition of occupation: ("doing things that are meaningful and purposeful") so that family members can understand why occupational therapy is named as it is.

Figure 21 is a photo of the downstairs powder room mentioned in the written case. Irene's son volunteers to change the sink and the mirror so that they are accessible, and the occupational therapist recommends standard equipment, such as grab bars. One approach would be to set up Irene's life on the first floor, and there is preliminary talk about installing a shower on the first floor. But Irene insists on being able to sleep in her own bedroom on the second floor. That is the room of her marriage, and it is full of symbols to her (Figure 22). She did not escape from the personal care home to be a prisoner of the first floor. To solve the problem, a stairglide is installed on the steps. A smaller wheelchair is donated for use in the narrow hallway upstairs. More modifications must be made to the upstairs bath, with Irene's son becoming skilled in the installation of mirrors and vanities. I want to stress that the occupational therapist gains the client's confidence by displaying both technical know-how and flexibility in problem solving. This trust will be necessary later when the therapist and Irene address sensitive cognitive issues. Hence, successful occupational compensations through home modification and assistive devices can enhance the therapeutic relationship so that occupational adaptation is later possible.

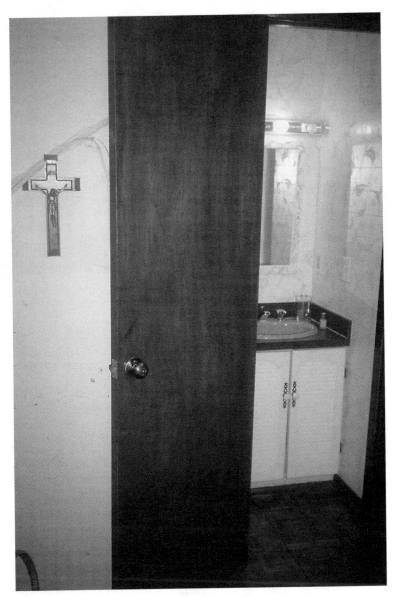

Figure 21. Simulation: Irene's downstairs powder room.

Intervention Outcomes

On the basis of your theoretical reference, what are the projected outcomes for this person?

Winnie Dunn
Ecology of Human
Performance

I was really glad when Dr. Law pointed out that she did not have any person–variable focus in her intervention; I think that we need to move away from such a heavy emphasis on person–variable interventions in this profession. I have special education and neuroscience degrees in addition to occupational therapy, so I know lots

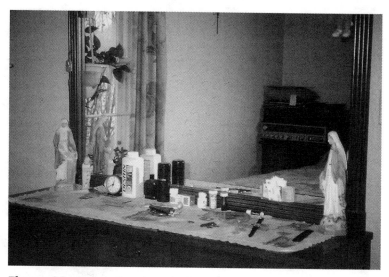

Figure 22. Simulation: Irene's dresser in upstairs bedroom.

Winnie Dunn

of evaluations, lots and lots of them. I know that I could test every one of you and find something wrong; for some of you, I would only have to be a trained observer to know your performance challenges.

How would you like to have to devote your whole day to work you do badly? Let's say you have a poor memory. Do you want to work on memory all day? How many of you use Post-it® notes? Post-it notes are adaptive aids to compensate for memory needs. Do I need to put you in a memory program if you use Post-it notes? I think that we need to think about the gifts of occupational therapy that we withhold from families when all we do is focus on improving person skills. Irene has the right to live her life; her son has a right to enjoy his mother. Some of our mothers who have not had an insult to their brains have poor memories anyway, and some of us have poor memories anyway. There is a point where families need our acknowledgment that the person is whole and can live a satisfying life regardless of memory (or any other) performance component challenges. We can think about a person's traits, just like being short or tall is a trait. We don't put you on a stretcher every night if you are "vertically challenged." We say, "Get a stool for the kitchen." We need to start giving the gift of making things available to people the day they want to do them. We need to be willing to do whatever it takes to support performance.

I think that in Irene's case, we have a history here where she has had some initial rehabilitation. She has had a lot of recovery time, and to continue to focus on those person-variables is not a reasonable approach. From an ecology framework, I would say that the outcomes that I would wish for Irene are related to finding a satisfying living circumstance. I recognize that we might have to go through some trials to find the proper mix of supports. For example, she might not like the personal care people who are available, and she might wish to choose some other ones.

At the beginning we tell the people that there are five ways that we try to solve their performance problem or desire. For example, we may not wish to take the cooking responsibilities away from Irene because she does it slowly since she likes cooking. So for me outcomes are related to doing a dance with this family to help them find the most comfortable pattern of supports that make Irene feel satisfied. This might mean that we need to find her a new place, making sure that her things are there so that it feels like her place. The outcomes for Irene and her son are focused on ways to make their lives satisfying again and how to reconstruct that in a way that is useful for all of them. We don't want to focus on her memory or her endurance problems by letting them interfere with her desired outcomes. We want to make memory and endurance issues as transparent as we possibly can so that Irene is competent to live her life. I think that sometimes we do not intend to send the message, but I think that when we focus on only person–variable outcomes, we continue to point out to the person that they are not competent. You know, "If you just were not mentally retarded we would be able to get this done." We don't say that, but this is the message that we send to families. Just as when we work with a person with spasticity, they may think that it is going to go away instead of thinking that it is part of who they are, and they can still have satisfying lives with that trait. At the stage of evolution of Irene's circumstance with her head injury, that occupational therapist needs to be supporting her performance desires.

Mary Law
Person–Environment–
Occupation Model

In terms of projected outcomes, our outcomes for Irene would reflect directly back to the issues that she has identified; that she wants to be able to do. The overall projected outcome would be that she lives with support at home. The support could come in a number of ways and is likely to come through a personal care worker or attendant care and instead of living in Toledo, if she lived in Toronto, she would have the option of managing the funds to hire her own attendant care worker over time.

Another important outcome for her is that she would be able to engage in a meaningful set of occupations that are chosen by her and are important to her. They particularly include leisure pursuits, which are obviously extraordinarily important to Irene. They were in her previous experiences, and there is no reason in the world why they would not continue to be. So when we are looking at this, we

Mary Law   need to look at how to structure her daily routine so that she has the energy and motivation to engage in these leisure pursuits. It is important that she does not expend her energy on self-care tasks that are easily done by someone else. Remember, occupational therapy does not equal activities of daily living.

I would also look for projected outcomes of changes within the environmental conditions in which she lives, in other words, changes in her home and in the community. Here we are looking at a much broader level so that any changes that are made, whether they are the church, the library, the neighborhood, would benefit everyone within these locations, so the focus is really on system changes rather than changes directed at the person.

In terms of looking at our accountability and our ability to say what Irene's outcomes are, the outcome measures that I would use would involve going back to the COPM and having her rerate the occupational performance issues that she initially identified. Other outcome measures that potentially could be used are the Functional Autonomy Measurement Systems (SMAF), and the Reintegration to Normal Living Index (Hebert, Carrier, & Bilodeau, 1988; Wood-Dauphinee & Williams, 1997). The Reintegration to Normal Living Index is an assessment that is very short but looks at her ability to reintegrate into the community in which she wants to live. The SMAF is a very interesting measure because it looks at independent living tasks and environmental resources in conjunction with each other. You can look at how changing environmental resources affects the tasks that she wants to be able to do.

David Nelson
Conceptual Framework
for Therapeutic
Occupation

Here is a somewhat different point of view concerning Irene's capacity to change (adaptation) and the occupational therapist's role. I do want to emphasize that CFTO does not necessarily require that the person changes; some occupational models of practice involve only compensation, not adaptation, and I respect this approach, especially if funding is limited. But in this case, I think that Irene has much potential to grow and to change. This commitment to adaptation fits in with the model of practice identified by Chapman (1996) (see Figure 23).

In occupational adaptation, the occupational therapist collaboratively synthesizes the occupational form that is meaningful and purposeful for the person. The person engages in an active, occupational performance resulting in adaptation; the person literally changes oneself through one's own act of doing (Nelson, 1994; Nelson, 1996). I think that this process of occupational adaptation is the reason that the profession of occupational therapy was originally invented.

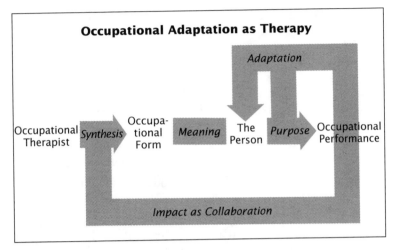

Figure 23. CFTO's depiction of occupational adaptation. *Note.* From "Why the Profession of Occupational Therapy Will Flourish in the 21st Century, 1996 Eleanor Clarke Slagle Lecture," p. 14, by D. L. Nelson, 1997, *American Journal of Occupational Thearpy, 51,* 11–24. Copyright 1997 by The American Occupational Therapy Association, Inc. Reprinted with permission.

So, let's not give up on Irene's ability to change her developmental structure through her own active occupation. We can posit sensorimotor change, cognitive change, and psychosocial change. Many people with traumatic brain injury continue to make gains for up to 5 years after the accident.

When we talk about projected outcomes, we are not just talking about movement for the sake of movement. We are talking about Sunday dinner at her house or an occasional celebration with the entire extended family at the Budapest Restaurant. We are talking about daily Mass at St. Stephen's, and Saturday nights at Tony Packo's. Other anticipated occupational outcomes include hockey games with her son and occasional trips to Hungarian stores and churches in Cleveland. Irene loves a good wedding, and the extended family is large.

To move forward on these goals, we are going to assume that Irene begins to attend a small, community-based occupational therapy center Monday through Friday, 10:00 a.m. to 1:00 p.m. We will also assume that a personal-care attendant is hired to assist Irene in the home. Practical things conducted in the therapeutic community can be integrated into Irene's daily occupations, and the therapist plans to work closely with the personal-care attendant so that therapy is carried over into the home. The therapist anticipates a problem of integrating a 70-year-old woman into a community of others with brain injury; most of the center's clients are young men, and

David Nelson

some have substance abuse problems that are foreign and potentially frightening to Irene. With the therapist's help, Irene finds a special role in helping to cook lunch. An occupational therapy student works with Irene and follows the occupational therapist's explicit instructions. Irene makes linzer cookies, plum dumplings, Hungarian hamburgers (made from pork), and tomato potatoes for "the boys" as she calls them. Cooking becomes the naturalistic context (part of the occupational form) for proper joint alignment, therapeutic guiding, and weight bearing.

The student also promotes cognitive adaptations by careful changes in the parameters of the occupational form in order to enhance specific cognitive processing strategies. The occupational therapist uses other naturalistic occupational forms to help Irene generalize cognitive processing strategies. For example, Hungarian church history is especially meaningful to Irene, so it serves as an excellent context for practicing memory strategies. (We identified a 10-page document listing events in Hungarian church history on the Web.) To ensure carryover into the home and community, the therapist works with Irene's son, her cousin, and the personal care attendant in designing forms to encourage cognitive strategies. For example, Irene's son learns how to help his mother engage in stimulus-reduction procedures at the first sign of agitation at the Budapest Restaurant or the Toledo Storm hockey game. Irene needs to learn how to ask for simple things, such as preferential seating. When confused by a menu, Irene learns to ask the waiter to come back after she has had a chance to think about it.

To ensure carryover of sensorimotor interventions, the occupational therapist instructs the personal care attendant to encourage Irene's weight bearing on the right scapula in supine-to-sit transfers and in morning self-care. The idea is to embed therapeutic movement within naturalistic, daily contexts. Irene needs to learn how to naturalistically elongate spastic muscles within the context of daily occupations. We are certainly not predicting return to totally selective movement of the right side, but these strategies will decrease the chances of impingement and pain in the right shoulder and right hip. Nobody needs impingement and pain, and it is something that Irene wants to work on.

The idea is to generalize, to her home and community, what she learns in the therapy center. Irene tries to return to her old role of reading stories to children, but the children have little tolerance for Irene's lack of cognitive flexibility. Adaptation is seldom a smooth process. Facing up to the new obstacle, Irene and her occupational therapist get the idea of volunteering at her former personal care home (the "old folks' home," as she calls it). There she reads stories on a regular basis to appreciative residents. They are very tolerant and appreciative of her method of reading stories.

Future Clinical Research
What future research questions are viable or needed to study clinical application of your work?

Winnie Dunn
Ecology of Human
Performance

To study the clinical application, I think we need to study the issues that occupational therapy had before us in terms of where our practice is going to be in the next 10 or 15 years. Additionally, when researching an area that already has been researched by another discipline, we need to bring the findings of that other discipline into the occupational therapy world to be considered. For example, I am going to tell you two stories that some of you have heard me tell regarding things that happened in the special education world during my early career that have a huge impact on choices about intervention. If you look at the EHP interventions—adapting, altering, and restoring—those are very important things for us to understand with choices that we are making with family. One of them is from the late 60s and early 70s.

In the late 60s it was very controversial to teach children with Down syndrome sign language because everybody thought that if we taught them sign language, they will never talk. From an occupational therapist's point of view, teaching sign language is an adaptation for talking. It is a way of working around the problem of oral communication. I was lucky enough to be in a setting where everybody was secretly sneaking signs with the children with Down syndrome. Of course, when children are young and have Down syndrome, you do not have to know very many signs. You know *eat, drink, potty, more, no* and *you are about done.* And kids with Down syndrome have low muscle tone so they do not make the signs very clearly. So I was in the throws of this controversy in my early career, and it was fascinating to me because what do we know now in 1999 about teaching kids with Down syndrome sign language? They do not get frustrated, they do not start having secondary behavior problems, they understand what communication is, and—guess what—*they talk sooner.*

The other piece of research that is important to this dialogue is in the middle 80s a series of studies were done with children who were nonmobile. People started putting these kids into electric cars. Everyone was upset about putting these kids who could not move into electric cars. Guess what happens when you put a kid who cannot move in an electric car? They drive away. They are thinking, "I've been carried around, I've been moved, I've been pushed,

Winnie Dunn

and now I'm driving away." They run into the walls and do all the same things the other kids do like our teenagers when they get into a car for the first time. But, what we learned from these series of studies is that when kids who cannot move are put in electric cars, and then we take them out of electric cars, *they move more.*

So here are two sets of studies that were done by people outside of our profession, a series of studies, which indicate to us that sometimes adaptation should be done first. I think that the historic tradition in our profession is that we do remediation first, and then when we realize that people are still going to have cerebral palsy, we give up and do adaptation. What I would like to see in terms of research is for our profession to start looking at what the conditions are under which adaptation should be done. What are the issues of the person feeling satisfied or feeling hopeful or what will he or she look to in the future if we give him or her access to doing things at the initial stages of the disability or crisis as opposed to waiting until he or she is through this recovery period.

In terms of what Dr. Nelson said regarding us making a difference, I think that focusing on the doing can result in changes. These two examples are exactly what he was talking about. You can focus on the occupation and have other person–variable changes as a result because of the person having access to the activity. So that relationship is something that would be very appropriate to study and might help us get away from always focusing on these performance component goals when, in fact, the goal is for them to be doing.

I think that those are the sorts of things that we need to be doing to inform us about how to make these decisions because we have an obligation to be telling families what their choices are, and what the evidence is about the choices that they are making. The evidence shows that if we do adaptations early, the person will be able to get back to cooking faster.

I also think that we do not do very well at giving families choices. We like to decide what the best plan is and we give it to them. So part of having more research available to us about these different choices gives us evidence to tell families, "Here are the things you might try." "This one is a little more risky." "We don't know what happens with this one." Creating evidence about adaptation and about how that process of adaptation helps the outcome the family wishes, I think would be important to the future of discipline development.

Mary Law
Person–Environment–
Occupation Model

I remember many years ago talking with an insurance adjuster about funding for an electric wheelchair for a 2½-year-old. The adjuster kept saying, "I have a 2½-year-old, and I would never put him in an electric wheelchair." I kept saying, "Does your 2½-year-old walk?" He said, "What happens if he runs into the walls?" I said, "You switch it off." I won that battle.

Before I talk about research questions, I want to give you some examples of some of the research that we have done to date with the PEO Model. It includes a critical review of the person–environment measures and studies of clinical utility of environmental measures. We also have a lot of work to do in terms of validating more environmental measures.

We have looked at the environmental factors that affect participation of children with disabilities, the effects of environmental sensitivity on occupational performance, transition to adulthood for adolescents with disabilities, and supportive work environments for people with persistent mental illness.

Some of the research questions that we think need to be addressed relate to how we get the "biggest bang for our buck" out of therapy. When do we intervene? What specific factors are the most important to make the difference in enabling someone to do the occupations that they want and need to do? We need assessments to tap the interface between person and environment and occupation to help give us that knowledge.

For Irene, what are the minimal levels of environmental support and personal support that will make the difference for her to be able to live at home and engage in the occupations that she wants to do? We also need an understanding of the critical periods. When do you intervene and when do you stop? Well, currently you stop when you do not get reimbursed anymore. Right? We have our own restraint, but it is at a higher level [Canadian health care]. You may only need to do one or two little things, and that may be the factor that makes the difference, or you may need therapy for a longer term. We really do not have that knowledge.

How does the person–environment relationship change over time? I'm thinking about this not only for persons who have disabilities and health issues, but for everyone. How does the relationship change over time as it ebbs and flows? How can this lead to development of new intervention strategies? For example, what about an increased focus on environmental intervention? What are the outcomes for that? We need to do studies related to that.

Finally, this relates back to what Drs. Dunn and Nelson have been talking about, does engagement in occupation lead to changes in performance components? I think it does, and I think that this is where we should be putting our emphasis right away. The rest will fall into place.

David Nelson
Conceptual Framework
for Therapeutic
Occupation

CFTO can be used as a template for categorizing, analyzing, and promoting occupational therapy research. If the essential act of the occupational therapist is to synthesize occupational forms, then it follows that the central concern of the occupational therapy researcher is to study the effects of synthesized occupational forms on performances, adaptations, compensations, meanings, and purposes.

The experimental analysis of occupation is one kind of research that I propose (Nelson, 1993). Here, the independent variable consists of two or more contrasted occupational forms. They are in the environment and can be manipulated. The dependent variable then consists of observable performances or impacts that can be measured objectively. Logical inferences are drawn about adaptations, meanings, and purpose.

One example of an experimental topic is the study of occupationally embedded movement. Here the independent variable involves a contrast between a naturalistic occupational form and a contrived (or rote) occupational form. This topic has become the first to be explored experimentally in any depth in our profession. I am sure that you are familiar with individual projects as well as the meta-analyses conducted by colleagues at Boston University (Lin, Wu, Tickle-Degnen, & Coster, 1997).

Other topics within the experimental analysis of occupation include (a) options and choice versus no options; (b) the opportunity for hands-on doing versus other forms of instruction, such as demonstration; and (c) different types of group structure. There are many other potential topics, most of which have been discussed as traditional principles of occupational therapy throughout the history of the profession.

CFTO is not restricted to an experimental approach. I am not a qualitative researcher, but I would enjoy seeing qualitative studies using CFTO. For example, Kielhofner and Barrett (1998) recently studied the relationships between occupational forms and the meanings of a woman in a vocational program in a Chicago inner city neighborhood. They contrasted the meanings of the woman with the meanings of the occupational therapist. I urge you to read that study. It should be noted that Kielhofner's definition of occupational form is slightly different from mine. However, the original definition would work just as well in his study.

Here is a quick recommendation. For qualitative researchers interested in grounded theory, you might consider using CFTO as the system of axial coding, as opposed to using the system outlined by Strauss and Corbin (1990).

My own research has shifted over the past couple of years from experimental analysis of brief occupations to the development of occupational assessments and the study of efficacy (the effects of longer-term occupational forms). CFTO continues to be an organizing framework for us as we develop truly occupational assessments for patients in skilled nursing facilities and subacute care and as we study the effects of occupationally based interventions on long-term outcomes. Today's case of Irene presents an excellent example of the kinds of things that I want to study: how the occupational therapist can facilitate the transition of someone like Irene from an institutional setting to her home, neighborhood, and family.

Janette Schkade
Moderator

Would you briefly discuss the relationship that you see among your theoretical point of view, education, and practice?

Winnie Dunn
Ecology of Human
Performance

I think that one of the things about the ecology framework that has been helpful, both for our faculty and our interdisciplinary colleagues who have worked on this with us, is that this framework invites people from other disciplines to join with us in looking at problems. We have the Center on Aging; Kansas University has a Pepper-Center grant which is a grant to study issues of older adults in honor of Claude Pepper; and the Center uses the ecology framework as one of their theoretical frameworks because it invites people from other disciplines to join together in solving some of these common problems.

We are also involved with the Center for Research and Learning in Kansas. They do a lot of federal grant projects. We just finished a project, for example, where we wrote an entire manual for people in adult education programs to include people who had ADA (Americans With Disabilities Act) needs and issues that were keeping them from doing work and keeping them from getting their GED (General Educational Development) diploma. The whole manual is written from the perspective where the problem that the person has is stated at the top and the ecology interventions are listed across. All the adaptations and restorative strategies that you might do for that problem are listed on the work sheet so that these adult basic educators can pull out the sheets and say, "Oh, there's another idea that I can use." We have a whole notebook that applies the ideas that come from occupational therapy problem solving to the problems that people in these other disciplines experience. We are now designing them for people who work in community college systems. We developed an evaluation for the learner. Now we will develop an evaluation for the teacher to evaluate the kinds of learners that would be consistent with your style and which kinds of learners would be more challenged by your style in terms of ADA outcomes. That is an example of taking this framework and taking it to a practice situation.

I think in terms of more occupational therapy practice; the idea that there are five different ways of looking at every single problem is a really useful link to practice. It gets us out of the "if you have this problem you do this, if you have this problem you do that." It helps you to see that if there is a problem, the person has the right to consider five ways to solve it. The occupational therapist then has the framework to come up with the different ideas and offer them to the family. It is a continual reminder that we have those options available to us as we engage in the practice of our profession.

Mary Law
Person–Environment–
Occupation Model

When we look at the implications for practice for the PEO Model, I think it provides a way and method that we can make certain that we consider the complexities of human functioning and experience. In particular, we need to consider occupational performance over time and within different environmental contexts. This model is a way that therapists can approach the analysis of occupational performance over time and to try to figure out what is helping, what is hindering, and where intervention should be focused.

It helps therapists to expand the scope of practice, particularly in terms of increasing our focus on environmental intervention, not just at the level of the person, but also at the level of the neighborhood community and system. We have found in our experience that it really is very useful in facilitating communication and, similar to Dr. Dunn's experience, we have used it in many multidisciplinary situations with clients, and with others as a communication tool to explain the focus of occupational therapy and to work out intervention plans.

Also, the model supports client-centered practice because you begin from where the person is and what they want to be able to do. As an example, Figure 24 shows you the temporal nature of Irene's experience over time. You get a flavor of her life as it was before the accident happened in July 1997 as far as occupational performance and congruence between person–environment and occupation. What happened at the time of the accident in November 1998 when we know her and in the future? It is a way of analyzing outcomes.

Here are some application examples of where this model has been used. It was used for development of a home support program in Baffin Island. It has been used in the development of rehabilita-

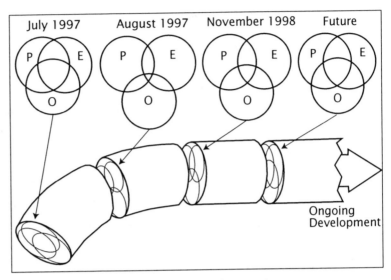

Figure 24. Temporal nature of Irene's experience.

tion programs in Bosnia. It served as a basis for an international, clinical fieldwork experience that two students from our facility had in India. It was used for career planning for occupational therapy students in New Zealand as a basis for school health students in Ontario, and it was used for workplace reentry. We have also used the model to develop a family-centered functional approach to children's rehabilitation. It was also used in the new practice guidelines for occupational therapy in Canada and for the blueprint for our national examination in Canada.

David Nelson
Conceptual Framework
for Therapeutic
Occupation

The CFTO's definition of occupation is very broad. Occupation is anything one does with meaning and purpose. The thing that is done is the occupational form. The doing is the occupational performance. A person might do something with minimal meaning and purpose, as we saw with Irene in the personal care home. Or, a person could be almost bursting with meaning and purpose, as you can expect Irene to be as she is going up that lift into St. Stephen's every morning. The CFTO defines essential concepts of occupational therapy and then states their relationships to each other. These include the concepts of culture, the nonhuman environment, objects, subjectively experienced meaning, perception, intrinsic and extrinsic purpose, measurable performance, adaptation, and compensation. Precise definition is important. Sometimes a word is used by one person, and communication with another person is assumed. This can be dangerous. For example, Dr. Dunn and I define the term "adaptation" in different ways. What she calls "adaptation," I call a type of compensation. What she calls "remediation," I call a type

David Nelson

of adaptation. I have reasons for using the term as I do, and I am sure that Dr. Dunn has her reasons also. The point is that many of the basic terms in occupational therapy are defined in multiple, contradictory ways. Therefore, a theoretical system must be very careful about definitions leading to clear communication.

Occupational therapy is a dynamic interactive process, and I think that CFTO depicts it as such. The founders of our profession of occupational therapy held absolutely passionate beliefs in the potentially therapeutic effects of occupation on the human being. Eleanor Clarke Slagle (1922) talked about a system of occupational analysis, and she talked about adaptation through occupation. I think that the occupational analyses and occupational syntheses of our students at the Medical College of Ohio are consistent with Slagle's insistence that we attend rigorously to the objective circumstances of the person as well as to the subjective experiences of that person.

In today's case of Irene, I tried to show how CFTO is compatible with an emerging model of practice that itself draws upon several other models of practice. CFTO is flexible across all the occupational therapy models of practice; it is a common language. So CFTO can be used with Kielhofner's Model of Human Occupation, or it can be used with a very different model of practice, such as Allen's Model of Cognitive Disability. CFTO can be used with sensory integration. It can be used with rehabilitation-based compensatory models.

In addition to the flexibility of CFTO, CFTO terms are immediately practical. For example, we have designed a system of writing narrative progress notes using CFTO terms. Instead of SOAP notes we call them SOAR notes. The "S" part is the synthesis of the occupational form–that is the therapist's plan. The second part is occupational analysis—"OA." That is the description of the objective characteristics of the person's occupation and an analysis of required component abilities. The "R" is the resynthesis of the occupational form–the plan for future intervention, given progress to date as described in the "OA" section. This system of documentation is simple, it is logical, and it is occupation-based. We have found that third-party payers and Medicare reviewers accept this system, to date. Who could blame a profession called *occupational therapy* for using the term *occupation* and other occupational terms?

I will conclude by repeating what I said in my Slagle lecture (Nelson, 1997). As soon as we become comfortable using occupational terms, the public, the payers, and our fellow professionals will become comfortable and appreciative of our unique services.

Audience Questions

Audience Participant

Have you ever shared your graphic representations of your framework with your clients because it struck me, listening and watching, that the relationships that these pictures portray would be very helpful to people in the problem-solving period. I think that if people can create a new picture, then often they can create the solution to do it. Of course, all of these diagrams have a lot of visual appeal to me, and I would think that for our clients and their family members, they would be very enabling and freeing kinds of pictures to help people see the relationships.

Winnie Dunn
Ecology of Human Performance

We give out buttons. To both our colleagues in other disciplines that work with us and to the families when they understand it well enough to get a button.

Mary Law
Person–Environment–Occupation Model

We have had quite a few experiences in using the model with clients and for programs, including the planning stages. The experience with clients has been very positive using paper models and we've actually tried to use some three-dimensional things as well. It is really hard to display three dimensions on paper, as you well know. But the model has worked very well because it is a visual tool that clients can see and use to look at the choices. For example, "If we do this, it will have the effect of moving the environment closer to improve performance." Or, "Let's look at what is happening to you right now. Why are these issues happening to you at this point in your life?" It might be that the occupation is pulling away or the person's skills are pulling away. This has proved to be very, very useful as a communication tool and to help with the understanding of the occupational process.

David Nelson
Conceptual Framework for Therapeutic Occupation

We work very hard to explain occupation to clients, and we work very hard at how to explain it to people with different kinds of cognitive and language abilities and to people from different cultures. We try to explain that occupation means to do things with meaning and purpose. So, in occupational therapy, the person helps oneself by doing things that are meaningful and purposeful, with the therapist as a helper. The diagrams presented in this talk, however, are meant for professionals. They are too abstract for most people who seek a beginning understanding of what the profession has to offer.

Audience Participant

Why is your model using the word *task* instead of *occupation* in the EHP framework?

Winnie Dunn
Ecology of Human Performance

One of our objectives is that our conceptual work would invite interdisciplinary colleagues to join with us. I have spent most of my career with people from other disciplines. When we wrote the EHP framework, our intention was to make it so that it had core occupational therapy ideas and principles, yet we invited people from other disciplines to join with us in solving the problems that we all face. The interesting thing has been that we have had people from other disciplines take this model and use it, as well as us, in their grants, and in their papers and project products. It has not diminished the contribution of occupational therapy because they do not say, "We're taking this and going home." They come back and ask us more questions. The gentleman from the Center for Research and Learning project, doesn't write any grants without putting occupational therapy in them. Now he is branching out and is asking other prominent occupational therapists to join on a project. He would not write a grant without occupational therapy. It isn't that he took our knowledge and went away. He took our knowledge and said that these people have a lot to offer. So, I think our purpose of writing the EHP framework was to invite others to join with us on our work and to think it does have a different purpose.

Audience Participant

I'm not as familiar with the models used in Canada except for yours as I heard about it most. Are there other models used in Canada and if not, do we in the United States think that we will have one unifying model in the future?

Mary Law
Person–Environment–Occupation Model

There are other models used in Canada. Our new guidelines which are published in the book entitled, *Enabling Occupation*, use the COPM and the Canadian Model of Occupational Performance (Canadian Association of Occupational Therapists, 1997) and the PEO Model as an analytic tool. Certainly, many of the models of practice that people use here in the United States are used in Canada as well. What the COPM and increasingly the PEO model are used for are a basis for education, practice, issues, papers from the national association, and a blueprint for the certification exam. This is an activity that has gone on for many years in our country in terms of developing guidelines. I think that it has enabled us to have a very coherent approach both to practice, education, and communication, particularly when we are communicating with government. So, it does not preclude the use of other models, but it is the basis from which we start. It does give us congruence. As to the second question, I will give you my opinion as a very interested outsider who spends quite a bit of time in the United States. I think that you could reach a point where you had a model or framework that could be used in a similar sense to the way that we use ours to frame how you communicate in occupational therapy and how you frame education. I think that you probably have the basis of that in some of your standards that you have developed. I do not think that precludes using other models. What I have observed at times, however, as an interested outsider, is a competitive aspect to this. The experience of developing a model and coming together to write guidelines that I have been involved in is an experience that ebbs and flows and inevitably ends up in a good compromise. In the United States, I have observed some competitiveness among different approaches that could potentially get in the way of such a process.

David Nelson
Conceptual Framework
for Therapeutic
Occupation

My perception of theory and model development in the United States is that the lively debates reflect healthy concern for the fundamentals of the profession. I think that what we have is a great situation. Diversity is good. Even if diversity of opinion were not good, we simply cannot pretend that there is broad consensus about many issues in occupational therapy. I am quite skeptical of doing theory by committee, with formal votes and compromises on theory. Students and others find real comfort in having uniform terms and voted-upon philosophical statements, and there is value in these statements as a starting place, or as a snapshot of where we stand at a particular moment. *However*, analysis of various AOTA position papers as approved by the Representative Assembly reveals multiple, logical inconsistencies as well as errors of omission. I do not think that we are really ready for consensus on the basic issues in the field; it is a natural time for ferment. So when I see active debates among scholars, each of whom is trying to maintain logical consistency and comprehensiveness, I am happy for the profession. We have a wonderful engagement going on, as we can see here today, and I would not want theoretical issues transformed into politically charged legislative motions.

I think the real problem with model development and uniformity relates to interdisciplinary issues. Theoretical models are being developed at the international level (i.e., ICIDH-2) (World Health Organization, 1998) and at the national level (i.e., the Rehabilitation Science Model developed by the Institute of Medicine) (Brandt & Pope, 1997). Although these models have definite value in promoting interdisciplinary communication, I am concerned that the federal government might force the use of nonoccupational interdisciplinary terminology in order for scholars to qualify for fund-

David Nelson

ing for doctoral programs or research grants. If all your doctoral study and your postdoctoral study take place in a transdisciplinary atmosphere, intradisciplinary concerns will diminish and intradisciplinary language will atrophy. This could snuff out our inquiry into the nature of occupation, at least in this country. I think that this is the most real danger to the infusing of occupation into therapy.

Audience Participant

I'd like the panel to address the issue of psychosocial factors in their models and how you might embrace those as well as including issues of emotion such as our case—the idea of loss of occupational performance.

Mary Law
Person–Environment–
Occupation Model

You would certainly look at psychosocial factors within each part of the analysis. So in terms of the person, you would seek information about Irene's sense of self; her view of disability which she, no doubt, held previously; and how that impacts her now and how that changes over time. Within the environmental aspect, you would assess the social and cultural environment including social attitudes and psychosocial issues and how that impacted on her ability and the supports that are provided for her to do what she wants to do. Within the occupation dimension, you would want to consider what are the psychosocial aspects of the occupations that she wants to be able to do, and how they are providing meaning for her.

Winnie Dunn
Ecology of Human
Performance

I think that the psychosocial, the person variables related to psychosocial performance, are heavily intertwined with the contextual variables, especially the social–cultural variables. They are also related to the physical environment and how people derive meaning from different things that are in their environment. I think that we need to deal with psychosocial issues as they intersect with the things the person wants to do and the places they need to do them. To me, that is where the psychosocial features unfold—either as supports or barriers to their performance.

David Nelson
Conceptual Framework
for Therapeutic
Occupation

Consideration of emotion and psychosocial issues is an inherent aspect of CFTO's format for occupational analysis. Affect always colors meaning and purpose: That is a basic premise of CFTO. In discussing Irene, I noted the importance of her fears of increased disability and death; her painful awareness of decrease in cognition; her frustration with limited mobility and pain; her boredom; her felt religiosity; her hope for life; and her desire to escape the personal care home and to go home to live. These are major meanings and purposes. I also talked about her little pleasures in life and even her vanities (like her feelings about cheap silverware) that the therapist becomes aware of in order to develop therapy goals as well as methods. Indeed, the reason that we went to all the trouble to invent the particulars of her life was to convey an overall portrait of an actual person, and all actual people have powerful emotions. The CFTO format identifies emotion-laden meanings and purposes as absolutely necessary to consider, and it sets up a whole framework for doing that.

Audience Participant

I heard that the focus of assessment from an EHP perspective is mostly related to the environment and the client's desires. I wondered if you felt like there was a place in your model for evaluation of some of the "p" issues like vision, executive function, even things like literacy so that you can recommend this range of accommodations or adaptations that will truly be client-centered and fit?

Winnie Dunn
Ecology of Human Performance

I think that perhaps in my comments I was focusing on the other features because I think that we have overemphasized assessing the person's component skills without ever considering what they want or need to do. I think that the only way to come up with appropriate adaptations or restorative strategies is by knowing the person variables. It is interesting because in different settings, occupational therapists have to use those skills more or less, depending upon what other team members have in their repertoire of skills. Certainly those are gifts that allow us to understand how to make the adaptations. We would certainly need to do that. That emphasis needs to be diminished a great deal when we go into a community practice.

Mary Law
Person–Environment–Occupation Model

It is certainly important to look at those key factors. I think the key issue is when you do it. So rather than beginning by assessing the person variables, you begin by finding out what the person needs to, wants to, or is expected to do. What are the occupational performance issues? That drives further assessments in terms of performance components and environmental conditions.

Janette Schkade
Moderator

I want to thank this panel for an educational experience. I think we have a richer understanding of how each of their perspectives has an effect on practice.

References

Americans With Disabilities Act. (1990). Pub. L. 101–336, 42 U.S.C. §12101.

American Occupational Therapy Association. (1994). Uniform terminology for occupational therapy—third edition: Application to practice. *American Journal of Occupational Therapy, 48,* 1047–1054.

Baum, C., & Edwards, D. F. (1994). Cognitive performance in senile dementia of the Alzheimer's type: The kitchen task assessment. *American Journal of Occupational Therapy, 48,* 431–436.

Brandt, E. N., & Pope, A. M. (1997). Enabling America: Assessing the role of rehabilitation science and engineering. Washington, DC: National Academy Press.

Bronfenbrenner, U. (1977). Toward an experimental ecology of human development. *American Psychologist, 32,* 513–531.

Canadian Association of Occupational Therapists. (1997). *Enabling occupation: An occupational therapy perspective.* Ottawa: CAOT Publications.

Chapman, L. M. (1996, May 3). *Traumatic brain injury rehabilitation: Promoting positive outcomes.* Workshop given at the Medical College of Ohio, Toledo.

Dunn, W., Brown, C., & McGuigan, A. (1994). Ecology of human performance: A framework for considering the effect of context. *American Journal of Occupational Therapy, 48,* 595–607.

Hebert, R., Carrier, R., & Bilodeau, A. (1988). The functional autonomy measurement system (SMAF): Description and validation of an instrument for the measurement of handicaps. *Age and Aging, 17,* 239–302.

Iwarsson, S., & Isacsson, A. (1996). Development of a novel instrument for occupational therapy assessment of the physical environment in the home: A methodologic study on "the enabler." *Occupational Therapy Journal of Research, 16,* 227–244.

Kielhofner, G., & Barrett, L. (1998). Meaning and misunderstanding in occupational forms: A study of therapeutic goal setting. *American Journal of Occupational Therapy, 52,* 345–353.

Law, M., Cooper, B., Strong, S., Stewart, D., Rigby, P., & Letts, L. (1996). The Person–Environment–Occupation model: A transactive approach to occupational performance. *Canadian Journal of Occupational Therapy, 63,* 9–23.

Law, M., Baptiste, S., Carswell, A., McColl, M., Polatajko, H., & Pollock, N. (1998). *Canadian Occupational Performance Measure* (3rd ed.). Ottawa: CAOT Publications.

Lawton, M. P. (1986). *Environment and Aging.* (2nd ed.). Albany, NY: The Center for the Study of Aging.

Letts, L., Scott, S., Burtney, J., Marshall, L. & McKean, M. (1998). The reliability and validity of the Safety Assessment of Function and the Environment for Rehabilitation (SAFER) Tool. *British Journal of Occupational Therapy, 61*, 127–132.

Lin, K., Wu, C., Tickle-Degnen, L., & Coster, W. (1997). Enhancing occupational performance though occupationally embedded exercise: A meta-analytic review. *Occupational Therapy Journal of Research, 17*, 25–49.

Nelson, D. L. (1988). Occupation: Form and performance. *American Journal of Occupational Therapy, 42*, 633–641.

Nelson, D. L. (1993). The experimental analysis of therapeutic occupation. *Developmental Disabilities Special Interest Section Newsletter, 16*, 7–8.

Nelson, D. L. (1994). Occupational form, occupational performance, and therapeutic occupation. In C. B. Royeen (Ed.), *AOTA self study series: The practice of the future: Putting occupation back into therapy, Lesson 2* (pp. 9–48). Bethesda, MD: American Occupational Therapy Association.

Nelson, D. L. (1996). Therapeutic occupation: A definition. *American Journal of Occupational Therapy, 50*, 775–782.

Nelson, D. L. (1997). Why the profession of occupational therapy will continue to flourish in the 21st century, 1996 Eleanor Clarke Slagle lecture. *American Journal of Occupational Therapy, 51*, 11–24.

Slagle, E. C. (1922). Training aides for mental patients. *Archives of Occupational Therapy, 1*, 11–17.

Strauss, A. L., & Corbin, J. M. (1900). *Basics of qualitative research: Grounded theory procedures and techniques.* Newbury Park, CA: Sase.

World Health Organization (1998). Towards a common language for functioning and disablement: The International Classification of Impairments, Activities, and Participation. Geneva, Switzerland: WHO/MSA/MHN/EAC/97.3

Wood-Dauphinee, S. & Williams, J. I. (1987). Reintegration to normal living as proxy to quality of life. *Journal of Chronic Diseases, 40*, 491–499.